HIIT

LOOK LIKE AN ATHLETE
FEEL LIKE AN ATHLETE
HOW & WHY HIIT WORKS

8 WEEK TABATA EXERCISE PROGRAM FOR BEGINNERS TO ADVANCED

NUTRITION PLAN

MEAL PLANS

SHOPPING LISTS

FOOD DIARY

Formulated By A Master of Science in Exercise and Nutrition Science, Bachelor of Science (hons) in Sports Science, Post Graduate Certificate of Education in Physical Education Specifically For The HIIT Program

by Steve Ryan

ISBN-13: 978-1530499946

ISBN-10: 153049941

#Disclaimer

It is important to understand that for a few people, high intensity exercise of any type can be dangerous. Consult your doctor before you begin any HIIT program as prevention is better than the cure. Even if you are fit and healthy it is often advisable to seek any advice from a qualified personal trainer when you are embarking on a new exercise regime.

Disclaimer and Terms of Use: Every effort has been made to ensure that the information in this book is accurate and complete, however, the author and the publisher do not warrant the accuracy of the information and text contained within the book due to the rapidly changing nature of science, research, known and unknown facts and internet. The Author and the publisher do not hold any responsibility for errors, omissions or contrary interpretation of the subject matter herein. This book is presented solely for motivational and informational purposes only. Consult your doctor before going on any diet or exercise plan. All of the information included in this book is intended solely for general and motivational information and should not be relied upon for any particular diagnosis, treatment, or care. This book is not intended to provide medical advice and is for general informational purposes only.

Contents

INTRODUCTION

Are you bored of your current training plan and feel that you're getting limited results? Or are you just beginning your fitness and health journey? Either way it is time to give '*High Intensity Interval Training*', or HIIT as it has become widely known, a real 'go' because it is a training system that is *scientifically* proven to work in terms of blasting off the fat, increasing your muscle mass, as well as reducing certain metabolic diseases.

The benefits of HIIT are actually well documented, and backed up with some robust scientific research. For these reasons HIIT has gained some real momentum in popularity over the last decade.

You may be thinking HIIT is just another training fad, and asking will it really work for you?

Well, HIIT will definitely work whether you are a beginner, a gym junkie or an elite athlete. HIIT is a powerful training method that gives you far quicker physique and health benefits regardless of your baseline fitness levels. Everyone will start to see quick and amazing results due to the effectiveness of this easy to follow training method.

HIIT is not complicated and you don't have to be a rocket scientist to add it in your current training program. Alternatively you can just start afresh and begin your HIIT journey right here!

With HIIT you can use as much or as little fitness equipment as you want, you can perform it at home or in the park, it takes less time, and you achieve rapid results in a fun and totally engaging way.

There are indeed many health benefits attached to this unique training method and all will be revealed in greater depth as we move through the book. Think of this book as a pocket guide and coach to HIIT training, and the following questions will be discussed in detail and answered concisely:

- What is HIIT training?
- What are the real benefits of HIIT training?
- What are the different HIIT training models?
- What is the science behind HIIT training?

After these four key areas have been discussed, it is then time to practice what we preach! In other words we have created a section on HIIT work outs along with a nutrition plan. These plans have been created by pulling together all of the relevant information from the previous 3 Chapters, this will help you to hit the ground running in terms of your fitness, health or physique goals when using HIIT. What are you waiting for? Let's get going!

ABOUT THE AUTHOR

Steve Ryan has a Master of Science degree in Exercise and Nutrition Science, a Bachelor of Science (hons) degree in Sports Science, and a Post Graduate Certificate of Education in Physical Education (Qualified Teacher Status). He has over 10 years of experience as head of a Physical Education department in a large British school. Steve has also been self-employed for 5 years; creating and implementing fitness and nutrition plans for private clients.

Steve helps with various individual needs such as weight management, gaining muscle mass/tone, improving athletic performance, enhancing cardiovascular health along with numerous types of mental & physical rehabilitation.

Steve specializes in medical referrals and obesity related issues; as well as being a strength and conditioning expert.

Steve has been prolific in writing educational resources, with over 700 under his belt, including exam questions, sport's coaching manuals, academic reviews, fitness/nutrition articles, training/nutrition plans and books and courses. He is passionate about the HIIT model due to evidence of the quick results, ease of fitting into busy lifestyles, and the many health benefits that ensue from it.

CHAPTER 1
WHAT IS HIIT?

High intensity interval training is defined as 'repeated bouts of exercise at maximal intensity, that reflect your peak VO2 maximum, with active rest intervals in between'[1]. VO2 max, or aerobic capacity, is the amount of oxygen consumption that you can uptake in relation to your bodyweight when exercising [1]. This system is very reliant on oxygen to convert energy into a fuel. However, HIIT training develops both the aerobic and anaerobic energy systems which is excellent news, as both systems have certain health and fitness benefits attached to them.

The ability to develop aerobic and anaerobic fitness in a single work out sets HIIT apart from traditional cardio and resistance training. It is this positive double whammy that makes HIIT so popular with fitness enthusiasts and elite athletes alike, because it combines both cardio and resistance training in one. You do have to train at a higher intensity but you will be performing the same or very similar exercises during HIIT e.g. the same push-ups, squats and lunges.

It is the change in exercise intensity combined with the duration of the lower intensity periods that are the key variables for unleashing the amazing benefits attached to HIIT training. The increase in exercise intensity is the main reason why you shred the fat, increase your muscle mass and improve your health goals. The mechanisms behind this will be discussed in Chapter 3.

You may be thinking how long should a HIIT session last? How many times a week can I perform a HIIT session? How are the work and rest interval timings related to my goals? Please read on and all will be revealed.

THE BASIC HIIT MODELS

High intensity interval training is an enhanced form of interval training that enables you to work for short bursts of high intensity activity followed by a lower intensity recovery interval.

These maximal bouts of high intensity exercise and the following lower intensity intervals can be adjusted to match your fitness levels. The fitter you are or become, the longer the bursts of high intensity activity.

A typical HIIT session lasts between 9-20 minutes, and these short intense work outs can provide improved athletic capacity, conditioning, improved glucose metabolism and fat burning potential[2].

INTENSITY OF A HIIT SESSION

When performing a HIIT session you will be exercising at a very intense rate during the high intervals. You will be near or at 100% of your maximum heart rate for short periods of time, and it is this strategy that improves both your aerobic and anaerobic fitness levels.

A basic HIIT model is made up of 6-10 high intensity exercises which are separated by a medium-low intensity exercise period. The number of repetitions and the length of each high and medium/low interval can be altered to suite your fitness levels.

The exercises can also be adjusted to suite your needs e.g. a repetition may include 20 seconds high knee sprints followed by 40 seconds jogging for recovery purposes. Your body will be in a high intensity state during the high knee sprints and in a lower intensity/recovery state in the jogging phase.

This sprint/jog repetition could be repeated 8-12 times during a training session but again this will be dependent on your fitness levels at the start of the program.

For the purpose of this book we will present the ratio of high intervals to low intervals as follows:

high intensity work rate time: lower intensity work rate time.

Using this example for a sprint to jog ratio, it would be

20:40 seconds

and/or

1:2 ratio.

If this is not clear at this point it will become very familiar very soon.

OPTIMAL RATIO FOR REST VS HIGH INTENSITY

The amount of time that you perform the high intensity and recovery intervals is all dependent on fitness levels.

Beginners would not want to exceed a 3:1 rest to work ratio. For example a good starting point is a 15 second sprint followed by a 45 second brisk walk. As the exercises become challenging, such as bodyweight or free weight exercises, then more recovery time is needed.

As you progress through a HIIT work-out program your ratios will change e.g. intermediate levels could be 30 seconds of sprinting to 30 seconds of jogging. This would be classified as 1:1 work to rest ratio. For the advanced a 2:1 work to rest ratio is the norm and the 4 minute Tabata model of 20 seconds sprinting to 10 seconds of rest is an excellent example of this. Needless to say that you can mix up the ratios and you can always adapt the intervals to your fitness levels. Once you have the experience of HIIT you will know when to change the work to rest ratios.

A key point to remember is that building a solid foundation using HIIT is paramount to the success of your fitness and health goals.

BEGINNERS

As a beginner in the world of HIIT you may be feeling a little daunted by the high intensity nature of the work outs. If you feel that you are not physically prepared to perform HIIT don't worry, a simple solution is to adjust the intensity of the exercises to match your fitness level. For example you may not be able to sprint for 20 seconds; so you have 2 options:

1. Sprint/Run at 70-80% of your Maximum Heart Rate (MHR) for 20 seconds and jog 40 seconds

2. Sprint for 10 seconds and jog for 30 seconds

Both of these strategies work, as you build up your fitness levels and prepare physically and mentally for a HIIT work out. Again this is the versatility of HIIT as you can tweak the duration of the exercise, the rest intervals and duration of the repetition to match your fitness levels.

For the beginner this is important, as it will keep you motivated and on track for achieving your fitness and/or health goals.

In terms of building up to a HIIT session if you are a beginner, it is advised to try to exercise at 70-80% of your maximum heart rate to begin with. Then try and add some short bursts of 100% maximal intensity e.g. sprinting in place to build up your body's tolerance to this style of training.

You will discover that you can work for a longer duration at 70-80% of your maximum heart rate when compared to exercising at 100% maximum intensity, during the high intensity work intervals. However, it is important to build up to working to100% maximum intensity during the work intervals, as this is when you start to push your body to its capacity and all of the benefits of HIIT begin to materialise.

A key point to consider is that when you exercise at an intensity of between 70-80% of your % maximum heart rate, your muscles still have the capacity to work for longer intervals and the low intensity intervals tend to be shorter.

This is a solid strategy for building muscle, boosting your cardiovascular and aerobic fitness, but it does not maximize your anaerobic strength and power. In effect training at a lower intensity doesn't completely deplete the muscles of their short term energy supplies and it is this switch from using oxygen (aerobically) to create/burn the fuel, to creating/burning the fuel without oxygen (anaerobically); is again a massive factor in the positive impact of HIIT. We will discuss the aerobic and anaerobic energy systems in more detail in Chapter 3.

For people starting off on their HIIT journey you may find that you can't last for 10 minutes. This is because your anaerobic strength has not yet built up. This is normal and don't feel frustrated and remember that HIIT is about quality and not quantity.

Even elite athletes struggle with 30 minutes of HIIT training and if you are training for longer than this duration then you are not training hard enough.

THE IMPORTANT FEATURES OF HIIT

The main concept of HIIT is that in order to work your body aerobically and anaerobically simultaneously, you need to have high intervals that are 100% of your maximum heart rate.

These high intensity intervals really don't have to be very long in terms of time. Many of the most challenging HIIT models and work out plans only have high intervals lasting between 10-30 seconds in duration.

The flip side to this is that working at 70-80% of your maximum heart rate, you will be exercising for longer at this prescribed lower intensity. Ultimately you will only be improving your aerobic fitness levels and not your anaerobic fitness.

Therefore the main underlying message of this book is that the high level of intensity associated with HIIT is the crucial element for you to get quick and fabulous results in relation to your goals.

The biggest difference between HIIT and other training methods is that you need to work at a maximal intensity. In essence you should be able to perform 10-30 seconds of maximal intensity regardless of your fitness levels.

If you are exercising for around 2 minutes without stopping then you are not performing HIIT. If you are performing HIIT properly then you really do need the lower intensity intervals to complete the next repetition with any conviction and gusto.

This recovery strategy is vital and it will definitely be needed as it will help you to reenergize, ready for the next repetition. Regardless of your fitness levels it is important to push through the repetitions and give it your all and then you will start to see the results a lot quicker.

Another key component of HIIT training is that it is a flexible training method which you can alter the exercise type to keep your body guessing and this creates 'muscle confusion'. One of the most important factors of HIIT is choosing the right exercise type or variations, as this can stop your body from plateauing.

This strategy will help you to reach your health and/or fitness goals a whole lot quicker because of the concept of surprise and waking up muscle groups that you are not used to exercising.

All of the work out plans in Chapter 4 will incorporate a large number and variety of exercises that can be used anywhere.

CALCULATING TRAINING AND RECOVERY HEART RATE ZONES FOR HIIT

A heart rate monitor and some simple mathematical calculations are a quick method of working out HR training and recovery zones whilst performing HIIT. HR training zones show you what is the optimal intensity to work at to achieve your goals; as every zone has its own unique benefits, physical/health outcomes and physiological implications derived from them.

Advice About Using % MHR And Training Zones

- Target heart rate calculations are an estimate only and should never be taken as an absolute.

- If you are beginning an exercise program using heart zone, work at the lower end of the training zone to start with e.g. 65% versus 75%.

- Please consult your doctor before starting a training program.

% Maximum Heart Rate	Training/Recovery Zone	Typical Exercise
50-65	1. Health Zone	A steady walk
65-75	2. Cardio Base Zone	Jogging
75-85	3. Cardio Zone	Running
100	4. High Intensity	Sprinting Tabata HIIT

Using % of Maximum HR to calculate training zones.

As mentioned earlier, heart training and recovery zones can be calculated by following these simple steps:

[(220-age) – Resting Heart Rate] x desired % for training + resting heart rate= Training Heart Rate.

Step 1- Maximum Heart Rate (MHR) = 220 - AGE (say your age is 30 years) = 190 BPM

Step 2- Find your resting heart rate = 50 BPM

Step 3- 190 – 50 = 140 BPM

Step4- Find the heart rate training zone (Cardio Base Zone 65-75%) =

140 x 0.65 = 91 BPM
140 x 0.75= 105 BPM

Step 5 -add the resting HR to find the training heart rate =

91+ 50 (RHR) = 141 BPM
105+ 50 (RHR) = 155 BPM

Thus, the training heart rate within the Cardio Base Zone for a 30 year old is between 141-155 BPM.

The above calculation is known as the 'Karvonen Method' (KM) and works on the principles of the person's conditioned state and fitness levels in terms of resting heart rate. The 'Karvonen Method' is an alternative training heart rate measurement to using the % maximal HR method (220-age)[3].

WHAT IS THE RATIONALE BEHIND THE 'KARVONEN METHOD'?

One of the main advantages of the Karvonen Method is that it provides narrower HR target zones than using the conventional % HR technique.

Resting heart rate can alter significantly, and this has a strong correlation with fitness levels / conditioned state of the individual. Therefore, the athlete will need to generate a higher heart rate when deconditioned, as opposed to when they are in good shape.

This is due to the improved efficiency levels of the heart; to pump blood around the body. Resting heart rate is also lower or slowed down in athletes compared to non-athletes, and the difference between the maximum heart rate and the resting heart rate is called the *maximal heart rate reserve.*

As an individual improves their Cardio Vascular (CV) fitness, their resting heart rate will drop, and their heart rate reserve will increase.

Maximal heart rate reserve = maximum heart rate - resting heart rate

The 'Karvonen Method' provides a usable, widely accepted guideline for using heart rate training zones, and one of the main advantages of using this method is that it provides narrower HR target zones than using the conventional % HR technique.

Also resting heart rate can be adjusted in accordance with fitness levels; which makes the technique more robust for using with HIIT. Therefore, baseline fitness and resting heart rate play a major role in the whole goal setting and training calculations process.

The *'Karvonen Method'* is regarded by many fitness professionals as the gold standard when planning / performing / evaluating heart rate zone performance levels.

TRAINING / RECOVERY ZONES

Zone 1- Health Zone (50-65% Maximum Heart Rate)

Goals:

- Improve general health

- Start of an exercise/fitness program

- Used as a warm up & cool down by competitive athletes

This zone can improve the ability of muscular and CV systems to recover from high intensity training sessions, and should be used as a warm up or cool down strategy.

A steady increase in heart rate during this zone can produce some general health benefits and will maintain heart health to some degree. However, getting to the next zone (Cardio Base Zone) as soon as possible is recommended for enhanced/improved cardiovascular health benefits.

Zone 2- Cardio Base Zone (65-75% Maximum Heart Rate)

Goals:

- Weight loss

- Improve fitness levels

- Use as a recovery zone

- Improves energy levels

- Produces a stronger immune system

This zone is known as the fat burning zone and the recovery zone (which is the intensity used to recovery between interval bouts of work). Individuals training in this zone who train without variation will initially improve their oxygen consumption, but in the absence of overload performance will quickly plateau.

To avoid plateau in your goals in terms of fat burning and performance, increase your duration, frequency or both. Increasing the intensity will place a new stress on the CV system and enhance CV efficiency and calories burnt.

This zone has the following physiological benefits:

- Builds an aerobic base critical for improving heart and lung capacity
- Improves the body's capacity to store & transport oxygen/nutrients to produce energy
- Improves blood supply, haemoglobin levels and blood volume
- Burns some fat

Zone 3- Cardio Zone (75-85% Maximum Heart Rate)

- Improves muscular endurance
- Improves muscular force
- Increases cardiopulmonary efficiency
- Enhances weight loss
- Improves the ability to remove lactic acid

This zone is close to the anaerobic threshold, where the body can no longer produce more energy for solely aerobic metabolism, so the amount of energy produced anaerobically increases.

The higher the intensity that the body can train at aerobically, the more calories will be burnt from fat, and less lactic acid is produced. One of the major outcomes of cardiorespiratory training is an increase in the anaerobic threshold and a greater reliance on fat as a fuel.

This is good news if your goal is to reduce % body fat and full body weight loss, as there is a marked increase in the calories used due to an increase in intensity. However, in terms of athletic performance similarly to training in Zone 2, staying in Zone 3 will lead to a plateau in performance.

Progressive overload with frequency, intensity, time and type of training will keep your goals on track and prevents boredom kicking in.

Zone 4- High Intensity Zone (100% Maximum Heart Rate).

- Higher athletic performance
- This zones makes you faster and stronger

Most athletes train at this zone for short bouts consisting of about 10-40 seconds at a high intensity. It advised to recover in Zones 1 and 2 for a prescribed amount of time dependent on your goals, then return to Zone 4 for more high intensity work.

This zone has the following benefits:

- Increases speed, power, metabolism and anaerobic capacity by repeatedly exposing muscles to the high intensity
- Improves resistance to fatigue
- Improves endurance and CV capacity
- Burns more fat due to the higher intensity
- Activates the 'after burn' mechanism.

LENGTH OF A HIIT SESSION

HIIT is an extremely effective and very convenient form of exercising. As mentioned previously you don't need a lot of equipment, space or time to execute this powerful work out.

In the modern age where everyone is rushing around and spare time can be a sparse commodity; HIIT can fit into your current lifestyle with ease.

Unfortunately people still believe in the old fashioned 'Bro-science' training strategies that you need to spend 2-3 hours per day in the gym to get your dream physique. This is a training strategy that is very out-dated - HIIT has blown this notion totally out of the water. With HIIT you don't have to train every day for lengthy periods of time!

Many professional physique models and bodybuilders tend to train for no longer than 1 hour on a daily basis. Research has indicated that for HIIT to be effective all you only need to train a maximum of 20-30 minutes, 2-3 times per week2.

In conjunction with this research, it is not recommended to undertake HIIT training more than 3 times per week, as this could have an adverse effect on health and fitness goals! Even elite athletes only use HIIT a maximum of 4 times per week because over indulging can cause muscle damage and over training.

You really need 48 hours rest in between your HIIT work outs. This is in comparison to elite athletes who only need 24 hours in between HIIT sessions because their body tends to recover far quicker than normal individuals. If you train on back to back days you are putting your body at risk of injury because you are not allowing the body time to heal itself.

Research suggests that post exercise damage may be caused by cortisol and increased usage of type 2 muscle fibres. This damage can be evident up to 48 hours post exercise and bearing this in mind the guideline of HIIT training 2-3 times per week is very do-able and should be followed.

However, for a fitness beginner, in the first 4 weeks of a HIIT program it is recommended that you start off training twice a week. Your body will gradually adapt to the intensity of the HIIT work outs and you will need to increase the overload to ensure that your progress doesn't plateau. With HIIT training it is important to remember that less is definitely more.

A key point to consider is that 'when you enter into the 'anaerobic threshold' you will be taxing your body to the max'. It is very important to plan your HIIT training properly - Chapter 4 has provided all this for you with some amazing work outs to follow.

PLANNING YOUR TIME

If you plan and manage your time effectively then performing for a maximum of 20-30 minutes, 3 times per week should not be an issue. You can perform HIIT anywhere and regardless of other time commitments - everyone should be able to find 20-30 minutes in their busy schedule. Where there is a will there is a way, and HIIT is about having a committed and determined attitude.

In terms of going to the gym, think about these pertinent questions:

- How long would it take you to travel back and forth to the gym?
- How long would you spend in the gym?

By the time you travelled on a round trip to the gym and spent 1 hour a treadmill and/or machine weights along you could have completed a 30 minute HIIT session.

We are not saying to give the gym as a miss, but HIIT can be performed almost anywhere and there are definite alternatives to the gym when training. *Are you starting to see the bigger picture yet?*

HOW MANY INTERVALS SHOULD YOU DO IN A WORK OUT?

The total amount of intervals has a strong relationship with the length of your high intensity intervals. Remember that your total HIIT work out should last between 20-30 minutes and this includes your lower intensity or recovery periods/intervals.

If your high intervals are lasting over 40 seconds as a beginner, then you need to reduce the time, increase your intensity and add more rest i.e. the 3:1 work to rest model you will perform at 10 intervals of HIIT every 10 minutes.

Realistically as you get fitter you should be looking to progress to 20 intervals of 15 seconds and the 1:1 work to rest model of 15 seconds x 20 intervals over a 20 minute duration.

THE BOREDOM FACTOR OF TRAINING

In addition, some gym work outs can be deemed as boring. Sometimes you go into the gym on auto pilot and perform the same old routine. Same old boring routine= same results! Many of the HIIT exercises are bodyweight, use free weights and really need very little equipment and space e.g. kettlebells swings, forward lunges, squats etc.

These exercises maximise your fat burning potential and you don't need treadmills, weights machines and cross trainers to get into shape. Remember that HIIT is all about the right intensity, and using the right type of exercise will keep you switched on, prevent boredom from kicking in and this cute strategy will keep yon on track for your fitness/health goals.

Fundamentally HIIT is all about the mental and physical challenge that keeps you engaged and before you know it you will be hooked!

STEADY STATE CARDIO vs HIIT

HIIT burns calories up to 24 hours post exercise!

Before we move onto Chapter 2 it is very important that HIIT is championed in comparison to steady state cardio! You may have performed steady state cardio session at a lower intensity (65-75% of your maximum heart rate) for a minimum of 45 minutes per day whilst jogging, cycling or marathon training etc.

These types of exercises at lower intensities require oxygen and are not reliant on 'anaerobic metabolism' to meet their energy demands. You can exercise for longer at lower intensities and due to this concept the effects on the body are totally different when compared to HIIT.

Conventional or steady state cardio is good for the following:

- Burning calories up to 1 hour post exercise
- Improves your cardiovascular fitness

However, research has indicated that HIIT training can burn calories up to 24 hours post exercise[3] and this has been attributed to the muscles working anaerobically. This is called the 'after burn' effect. Training with HIIT 3 days per week, will give similar calorie burning results as performing a steady state cardio session for 6 days per week. You are saving time with HIIT and the impact of the 'after burn' effect is equivalent to training 6 days per week.

In addition, HIIT develops muscle tissue and explosive strength. This is also important in weight loss and maintenance as muscle is 15 times more metabolically active than fat and a constant supply of energy is required to sustain the life of the muscle. All of these metabolic benefits will be discussed in Chapter 2.

References

(1) Sharon A. Plowman, Denise L. Smith (2013). Exercise Physiology for Health Fitness and Performance. Wolters Kluwer Health

(2) Wilmore, J.H., Costill D.J., (2009) Physiology of Sport and Exercise. Human Kinetics, Champaign, Illinois.

(3) Powers S. Howley J. (2011). Exercise Physiology: Theory and Application to Fitness and Performance. McGraw-Hill Education

(4) Talanian JL[0], Galloway SD[1], Heigenhauser GJ[2], Bonen A[3], Spriet LL[4].Two weeks of high-intensity aerobic interval training increases the capacity for fat oxidation during exercise in women.[5], J Appl Physiol. (2007)

CHAPTER 2
THE BENEFITS OF HIIT

This Chapter will discuss the physiological and non-physiological benefits that are associated with HIIT.

You will be surprised how versatile and easy to perform HIIT actually is - the benefits linked to this unique training method are vast.

Some of the key benefits, such as being time effective, getting quick results and the fact that it can be performed at home or in the park have been discussed in Chapter 1. However, these topics will be explained further now, along with the health and fitness benefits, such as the reduction in body fat and the increase in muscle mass.

HIIT SAVES TIME

Reach your fitness and health goals in HALF the time with HIIT training.

As mentioned in Chapter 1 HIIT most definitely does save you time!

For the maximal effect and benefits associated with HIIT it is recommended that you exercise at this intensity for a maximum of 30 minutes per session, 3 times per week[1].Therefore it is easy to slot 30 minutes into your schedule and the excuses related to poor time management should be a thing of the past. There is evidence to suggest that 3 x 30 minute HIIT sessions has the same 'after burn' or fat burning potential as exercising at a steady state for 5 x 60 minutes per week[2].

In essence you are reaching your fitness and health goals in half the time with HIIT training. *What are you waiting for?*

THE 'TABATA' MODEL will save you time!

Tabata is the HIIT model which is the new kid on the block in the fitness world. The main reason why this fitness system is changing the way that we work out is quite simple - it takes a reduced amount of time to get rapid results in fat loss and fitness levels.

Dr. Tabata is a Japanese scientist who pioneered this training model whilst performing research on some elite speed skaters. He discovered that exercising at an intensity of 170% of your VO2 max (milliliters of oxygen per body weight per minute you can utilize) for 8x20 second bouts of exercise with 10 second rest intervals in between, had significant improvements in both anaerobic and aerobic fitness levels[3].

Let's breakdown a few points:

- V02 max (or aerobic capacity) is the amount of oxygen consumption that you can uptake in relation to your bodyweight when exercising. This system is very reliant on oxygen to convert energy into a fuel.

- In contrast, anaerobic fitness is your body's capacity to fuel its energy systems without oxygen and is important in sprinting and lifting heavy weights.

The research lasted for 6 weeks and the control group whom exercised at 70% of their VO2 max had improvements in their aerobic capacity but no improvement in their anaerobic fitness levels.

It is this improvement in your anaerobic capabilities that Tabata training produces; this facilitates increased fat loss and improved fitness levels.

THE TABATA MODEL

A Tabata model is as follows:

- Each exercise lasts for a duration of between 20 to 50 seconds

- After each exercise there is a 10 second rest interval

- Each round in Tabata lasts for 8 exercises

- Each round lasts for roughly 4-5 minutes

- You can stack the rounds to make a Tabata work out e.g.

  o 16 minutes = 4 rounds of 8 exercises lasting for 20 seconds with 10 seconds rest intervals in between.

Basically, you work at 110% in terms of effort, at a very high intensity for the allocated time (20-50 seconds) and then you rest for 10 seconds.

This will optimise your fitness goals; you will sweat your butt off because all of the exercises use large muscle groups and are compound in nature.

This enhances the quality of the session by improving metabolic conditioning, blasting up your metabolism and ensuring that your body is at its optimal fat burning potential.

A HIIT Tabata model will definitely strip away that dreaded fat - and the results are amazing.

Research has indicated that a Tabata style work out of 6-8 high intensity exercises ranging from 20-50 seconds (with a 10 seconds rest intervals) can burn up to 10 times as much as conventional cardio in a shorter period of time.

All of the exercises in the work outs should be performed with maximum effort i.e. move your butt at 110% effort pace! Your weight will definitely drop off and both your aerobic and anaerobic fitness levels will increase dramatically.

The question is why? This style of training increases your testosterone levels, enhances your muscle oxidation markers in your mitochondria (powerhouse of the muscle) and enlarges the muscles size and its overall power. This is excellent news especially as you are trying to gain overall body strength, increase muscle mass and lose the fat.

A key point to remember is that muscle is more metabolically active than fat, which equates to you burning more fat when resting[4]. This is all good news because you will be burning fat when watching television, sitting down in front of the computer and / or socializing with friends. Alcohol free of course!

Testosterone is a fat burning hormone which will give you a lean and healthy look. In addition Tabata training has the following benefits[3]:

- It boosts human growth hormone which is another major player in maintaining lean body muscle. Again please don't panic as growth hormone is a very powerful fat burner.

- Enhanced insulin sensitivity which is important for driving the glucose into the muscle and not storing the unwanted body fat.

- Burns fat up to 24 hours post exercise and uses fat stored as fuel.

- Improves muscle and liver usage of glucose which is an important body fuel.

- Boosts catecholamine levels that are required for the metabolism of fat.

- Preserves lean body mass which has been attributed to the anabolic effects of Tabata.

HIIT CAN SAVE YOU MONEY

Unfortunately many people use the excuse of have limited funds for not working out. Gym memberships can be very expensive, and if not sourced properly many home fitness products can be over-priced. It is this dilemma that many individuals find themselves in and these can be used as a barrier to exercise.

You don't need a gym membership to perform HIIT; as many of the work outs in Chapter 5 can be carried out at home, in a hotel room, or at the park.

If you live in a cold climate such as the UK, then another option is to maybe join the gym in the winter months and then cancel your membership during the summer. This strategy will save you money in the long run, as you can perform HIIT outside in the summer. However, you might be hard core and like to train outside in the winter or you are happy blasting through the HIIT work outs in your front room. Either way you will save money in the long run! Ultimately you will be getting a lot more 'bang' for your buck with HIIT!

YOU CAN USE AS MUCH OR AS LITTLE EQUIPMENT FOR HIIT

HIIT can save you time and it is also very convenient because you really don't need any equipment to perform it effectively. Some of the work outs in Chapter 4 only use bodyweight exercises and very little equipment and they can be performed almost anywhere!

If you want to pick up a few pieces of equipment needed for the work outs in Chapter 5, they can all be sourced very cheaply on the internet and ebay is probably a good place to start with. Try to buy equipment that will last and is not too flimsy, as you want to get your money's worth. It should at least last you throughout the workouts in this book and beyond.

Another key point to consider is that HIIT is not all about sprinting, although it can be an integral part of any HIIT regime. The good news is sprinting doesn't have to be included at all into the HIIT work outs. If you are not a big fan of sprinting then you can perform HIIT without it and use alternative exercises such as skipping, cardio hooping, agility ladder work and even sprinting on a home exercise bike. This is very good news! Try to remember that the gist of HIIT is all about the high 100% intensity and that the majority of exercises with or without equipment are meant to be very explosive!

HIIT is only really limited by your imagination, so make it fun and this will keep you motivated through the high intervals of the sessions. This is where you really need to push yourself - towards your capacity and beyond! This strategy will also prevent boredom - it's true what they say; 'variety is most definitely the spice of life'.

In terms of fundamental equipment needed to perform HIIT effectively you will need a good pair of running shoes, some comfortable training gear and a HIIT timer on your phone. Many of the apps are now free; so just shop around and find one that you can input your HIIT timing splits into e.g. 40 seconds higher intensity and 20 seconds lower intensity for 8 rounds etc.

HIIT AND SPORT

We have established that sport HIIT can be performed using a vast variety of different modes of exercise. This factor is extremely useful for anyone playing sport either on a professional or amateur level.

Many of the top athletes and sports teams use HIIT as an integral part of their preparation for their specific sports. The following section will highlight how HIIT can improve the athletic ability in a number of different sports. It also will summarise some of the major research findings relating to the sports in the table below (please use this as a reference to your specific sport):

Sport	Impact of HIIT on performance	Reference
Soccer	• Increases VO2 max in both man and female soccer players • Improves speed and endurance pre and post season • It improves speed, explosive power, strength and endurance • Prepares you for game play and enhances leg power which is an advantage when kicking the ball	5,6 & 7
American Football Rugby League Rugby Union	• HIIT used in off and during the season to improve lower leg strength, speed, vertical jump and leg drive.	8,9 &10
Basketball Volleyball	• Used to improve aerobic and anaerobic fitness • Improves your vertical leap and leg power • Improves explosive power when jumping	7 & 11
Cycling	• Improves the cyclist's VO2 max and anaerobic fitness • Improves fat metabolism, leg speed and leg power	12 & 13

A breakdown of the majority of sports

If you focus on the breakdown or composition of most team and individual sports they generally consist of short explosive high intense intervals followed by either a lower intensity interval or a rest.

Many of the professional and amateur teams and/or individuals are moving away from traditional cardio and using shorter and sharper HIIT sessions as a better substitute. A good example of this is in professional football where the sprint distances and times have been reduced in order to resemble real game time, as this is far more beneficial than running endless laps around the pitch. The whole mind-set has changed for the better for many sports and adding HIIT has its own unique benefits attached to it (see table above)!

Another trail of thought is that even endurance events such as the Tour de France and the London Marathon have short intervals of sprinting e.g. hill climbing or sprinting to finish the race. HIIT has started to become a staple part of the athlete's and cyclist's training and preparation plan.

Many athletes can now starting to train a whole lot smarter as they are starting to see the benefits associated with HIIT in a far shorter space of time than performing boring conventional cardio.

This strategy helps the individual to stay focused and the buzz attached to HIIT is far greater than steady state cardio.

HIIT BUILDS ANAEROBIC AND AEROBIC STRENGTH

As mentioned briefly in Chapter 1, HIIT improves both your anaerobic and aerobic strength at the same time. A study investigated the impact of a 6 week cycling program at an intensity of 80% VO2max in males. The cycling lasted for 27 minutes with a 1:2 work to rest ratio and it was performed three times per week. Even at an intensity of 80% VO2 max there were significant increases in both anaerobic and aerobic strength.

Bear in mind that HIIT should be performed during the high intervals at an intensity of near 100%, then you should get the notion that HIIT could further improve both of these fitness parameters. By increasing your anaerobic fitness you are enabling your body to perform at a higher capacity without oxygen and this is also vital to ensure the delay of fatigue.

HIIT challenges your fast twitch muscle fibres and it this mechanism that increases the size and strength of the skeletal muscle. The explosive and compound nature of HIIT resistance training recruits and challenges more fast twitch muscle fibres and this is one of the main reasons behind muscle and strength gains.

HOW HIIT INCREASES ATHLETIC ENDURANCE

Interestingly one of the major benefits of HIIT is that is actually boosts your athletic endurance. This is an unbelievable feat because HIIT's main features consists of short and explosive movements and many people associate endurance as being longer periods of time.

Typically the higher your VO2 max the better athletic endurance that you will have. VO2 max is a measure of maximum oxygen utilization of an individual during intense exercise. The higher a person's aerobic fitness, the higher their ability to consume and use the oxygen within the body when exercising. It is the body's upper limit for consuming, distributing and using the oxygen for the production of energy[14].

HIIT can improve your VO2 max and this is an excellent indicator of aerobic fitness. The concept of VO2 max is the ultimate marker for your cardiovascular health and fitness.

It is the concept of increasing and decreasing your heart rate to match the intensities of HIIT that creates a metabolic demand that actually improves your VO2 max. This is backed up by some valid research[15]; wherein it was discovered that after 15 weeks of a HIIT program there was a 12% increase in VO2 max and an improvement in power capabilities during the late and early stages of some power endurance tests. These results indicate that not only was there an increase in VO2 max, but power was maintained throughout the duration of the event; proving HIIT to be an excellent training method for finishing strongly during an endurance race.

Another trail of thought is that during a HIIT session your muscles are being taxed to the brink of their capacity and therefore require more oxygen. Training at such high intensities that closely mirror 100% of your VO2 max means that your body is reaching its 'anaerobic threshold'.

Theoretically this will improve your circulation, improve the efficiency of your heart at higher intensities and the mitochondria's size and number in the slow twitch muscle fibres increase with HIIT[14]. Hence your VO2 max will increase because of the body's improved efficiency at delivering and dealing the oxygen at a muscular level and this translates to improved endurance.

A review of the HIIT research on aerobic performance [16] concluded that six sessions of 30 seconds of sprinting over a 2 week period resulted in the doubling of endurance time to exhaustion. This was coupled with an improvement in muscle oxidative potential and it was identified that sprinting can boost performance in predominately endurance events.

THE HEALTH BENEFITS OF HIIT

WEIGHT LOSS

Losing weight by burning fat is possibly the biggest benefit that most people will be interested in. If burning fat is your main priority then you could not have picked a better mode of exercise.

The biggest difference between HIIT and other forms of cardio is how many calories that you burn *after* you exercise. When you have completed your HIIT session your body continues to burn calories whilst it is recovering from the high intensity

In essence HIIT turns you into a fat burning machine. In fact when you compare HIIT to other low intensity exercises, HIIT has been shown to be 50% more effective[17]. The 'after burn' effect and the science behind fat burning is explained in further detail in the next chapter.

A HIIT work out completed 20 minutes x 3 times a week is far more effective than exercising at a steady state for 40 minutes x 6 times a week. That is a massive difference in time and fat burning potential.

A key point to consider is to burn off 1 pound of body fat you must burn between 3,000-3,500 kcals. (This figure is dependent on your age, current BMI and genetics etc). HIIT boosts your metabolism when at rest, post and during the actually exercise and it is this mechanism that burns more calories compared to steady state cardio.

Let's use and breakdown the following example to make this valid point clearer:

- For argument's sake you burn 1000 kcals post exercise and with HIIT you will burn twice as many calories

- This equates to an extra pound of body stripped per week using HIIT as you will be burning an additional 3000 kcals

Interestingly to burn 3000-3500kcals per week you will have to perform steady state cardio for between 5hrs and 30minutes to 6 hours per week. This is a massive difference in not only time but the amount of body fat that is shifted between the 2 training methods. HIIT wins hands down over conventional cardio!

OBESITY

HIIT helps you to fight the fat but 'why is obesity such a health issue?'

The combination of being sedentary and poor eating habits can lead to obesity, and according to the National Health and Nutrition Examination Survey in 2010, the prevalence of obesity amongst US men was 35% and 37% for US women.

Three studies in the Lancet journal confirmed that obesity has doubled in the last 30 years, and 343 million men and 458 million women worldwide were now overweight / obese, and body mass indices and waistlines had increased vastly. It was reported that the fat are getting fatter, and that experts are warning of a tsunami of cardiovascular diseases and musculoskeletal injuries within the Western world.

Obesity increases the risks of high blood pressure, type 2 diabetes, stroke, sleep apnoea, gall bladder disease, respiratory problems, colon cancer and CV disease. This weight gain around the middle coupled with pressure placed on your joints and a weak core definitely compounds lower back pain.

Many people believe that by exercising a specific area of the body, the fat in that area will be utilized, reducing the locally stored fat. Results of several early research studies tended to support this concept of spot reduction. However, later research suggests that spot reduction is a myth and that exercise, even when localized, draws from almost all of the fat stores of the body, not just from local depots.

Combining HIIT cardio and resistance training blasts fat from all regions of the body, especially belly fat and around the core! This is good news because fat deposited within the abdominal area poses real health risks and it is associated with high insulin levels, increased cortisol levels (this is a hormone secreted when stressed) and poor sleep habits. Reducing stress and having a good night's sleep is an excellent combination when undertaking a HIIT program to reduce your body fat!

MUSCLE MASS

Many bodybuilders and physique athletes are big fans of HIIT. Many of these individuals who now use HIIT as a part of their training regime were in the past scared off by cardio as they felt that it blunted their muscular development and actually burnt away muscle mass. It was discovered that when bodybuilders performed conventional cardio for long periods of time there was a reduction in muscle development, and this was attributed to decreased levels of testosterone.

On the other hand HIIT can be a catalyst to improve muscle mass via increased levels of the muscle building and fat burning hormones. The science behind building mass is explained in further detail in the next Chapter.

A good example of HIIT in action is the difference in physiques between an Olympic sprinter and a marathon runner. Olympic sprinters are shredded with a very muscular physique and with minimal fat and marathon runners tend to be much slighter looking.

Sprinters work on explosive sprinting drills and this type of exercise is 'anaerobic' much the same as HIIT. This type of exercise actually facilitates the creation of muscle tissue and it burns fat. These short explosive intervals are an excellent platform for sprinters.

Conversely marathon runners need to conserve energy, pace themselves and they usually run at a lower intensity over a longer duration of time. Next time you log onto the internet punch in a marathon runner and a sprinter into a search engine and see the difference in physiques between both sets of athletes for yourself!

The Importance Of Sustaining Muscle Mass Through Life

HIIT resistance training improves glucose absorption in the muscle tissue; this action lowers your blood glucose and blunts the spikes in insulin. Boosting muscle mass can improve your energy production and its metabolic function and these are two key areas in health maintenance.

Muscle is more metabolically active than fat and research has indicated that individuals who performed HIIT over a 2 month period gained at least 2 pounds of muscle and lost 4 pounds of fat. This was attributed to the muscle's ability to rev up your metabolism at rest, and remember, muscle really does need a source of energy to survive i.e. burning calories!

As we get older our muscle mass is reduced between the ages of 35-75 years[17]. The American Council on Exercise reported that this was attributed to a loss in strength and the inactivity of the fast twitch muscle fibres. These fibres are activated during a HIIT session as they increase explosive power and strength. If your muscle mass is reduced, so is its capacity to absorb blood glucose and control insulin levels.

This stresses your pancreas and increases the likelihood of certain metabolic conditions e.g. type II diabetes. By adding resistance into your HIIT training plan it can have the following key benefits[17]:

- Enhanced quality of life because of a boost in your muscle strength and power

- A higher resting metabolic rate because of an increase in muscle mass

- Enhanced glucose tolerance, insulin sensitivity and an increase in the fat burning hormones

- A reduction in bad cholesterol and blood triglycerides and an increase in the good cholesterol

- Improved posture and overall joint health.

INSULIN

DIABETES AND THE ROLE OF GLUCOSE

The higher the amount of insulin in your blood, the more likelihood it will be stored as fat

HIIT lowers the amount of insulin that is released which is essential for fat loss.

Research has indicated that HIIT can have a positive impact on type II diabetes because of improved glucose control. It was concluded that performing HIIT 3 times per week improved average glucose levels 24 hours post exercise and that after 2 weeks there was a significant boost in blood glucose control[19].

Fundamentally, HIIT lowers the amount of insulin that is released, and high levels of insulin reduce your overall ability to burn fat. A key point to remember is that insulin's main role is store glucose so that it can be used as energy; ultimately this glucose turns into body fat if it is not used by the body as energy- this is a very valid point!

Excess glucose is not needed immediately by the cells and it stored as glycogen in the liver and muscle cells. Glycogen can be converted back to glucose when it is needed by the body as ATP (energy transfer) for muscle contractions and fuel for the brain.

You should think of insulin levels in your body as a measure of fat storage. After you eat a carb rich meal, your body converts these carbs into glucose and after digestion the glucose is transferred to the cells via your blood. Insulin promotes your cells to capture the glucose from your blood and this mechanism brings the blood glucose levels back into normal range.

For most individuals the amount of glycogen your body can store can range between 400-600 grams and the storage space is limited[17]. This is where fat comes into play - if your body is at its limit of glycogen storage, the excess glucose is stored by the body as fat. This is the main issue of 'insulin resistance' - that you need a lot more insulin to maintain blood sugar levels.

In a nutshell the higher the amount of insulin in your blood stream to deal with the glucose after a carb meal, the more likelihood that it will be stored as fat if the stores are already full! HIIT can actually improve your insulin sensitivity which is essential for fat loss.

In a study of non-diabetic and type II diabetic subjects, after 2 weeks of HIIT there was an improvement in fasting insulin and insulin sensitivity in both groups[19].

CONTROL YOUR CARBOHYDRATES

Another method of controlling your insulin levels is to consume less carbs, especially if you suffer with type II diabetes. However, if you are performing HIIT, reducing your carb intake may not be an option because you will definitely need the fuel. If you do increase your insulin sensitivity via HIIT, you can eat adequate carbs as an energy source without a huge spike in your insulin levels.

For obvious reasons you want to keep your insulin levels low to prevent fat storage. This means that you can eat healthy carbs whilst doing HIIT and still loose fat. For the record this scenario is a win-win situation for both diabetics and non-diabetics alike!

In addition HIIT reduces your blood pressure, increases your good cholesterol and decreases your bad cholesterol along with the blood triglycerides. These factors often go hand in hand with being overweight or obese.

HIIT STRENGTHENS YOUR HEART

HIIT is actually a great method of strengthening your heart because it ensures that blood is pumped to the lower and upper extremities in one repetitive cycle. It is this unique stress on the heart's function to meet the demands of HIIT that creates some amazing benefits.

The heart is essentially a muscle and needs to pump very hard to match the 100% intensity required to perform HIIT. During this 100% peak the heart's muscles will respond to this increase in demand and will in time strengthen.

HIIT is one of the best methods of strengthening your heart. It will adapt to periods of high intensity and cope with the stress of HIIT after just a few weeks of training. This has been backed up by the following research:

- A Swedish study reported that 4 rounds of 4 minutes runs at 95%HRmax performed 3 days per week for 8 weeks resulted in a 10% improvement in stroke volume[20].

- Another study noted that HIIT increased left ventricle heart mass and increased heart contractibility by 10%. The left side of the heart pumps blood around the body and the heart contractibility is related to improved cardiac muscle strength.

This increase in the capacity of your heart muscle will result in some major health benefits, such as an increased circulation, which reduces stress on the heart; along with lowering the risk of cardiac and metabolic diseases.

A Norwegian study investigated whether the intensity of the exercise decreased chances of cardiovascular mortality[21]. The study had over 50,000 subjects and after a 16 year follow up it was concluded that performing high intensity exercises once a week reduced the risk of cardiovascular death in both sexes compared to sedentary individuals.

This was backed up another study which concluded that HIIT is a time efficient means of improving cardiovascular disease risk factors in adolescents[22].

A good circulatory system is absolutely essential to us all for health throughout all stages of our life, and the body needs sufficient oxygen to be delivered to each cell. In addition good circulation ensures the body gets all of the vital nutrients and that all toxic waste is removed more effectively.

Why not give HIIT a real go, as maintaining or improving your heart's health is definitely the way forward!

MAY EXTEND YOUR LIFE

The positive impact and the associated benefits of HIIT can actually help you to live longer. This is backed up by a 4 year Harvard University study on 17, 000 males that concluded that only high intensity exercise and not moderate exercise reduced the risk of death[23].

HIIT has the following amazing benefits that will reduce the risk of death:

- It increases your peak oxygen uptake and this ensures that you stay fitter for longer and that there is no decrease in your functional fitness e.g. walking up stairs and/or carrying the shopping with no issues.

- It reduces body fat and insulin resistance - two factors which are associated with high incidents of metabolic diseases and an increased chance of mortality.

FUNCTIONAL FITNESS AND HIIT

FUNCTIONAL TRAINING

Over the past decade, there has been a shift in making training more functional. The revolution started with physical therapists and filtered its way into personal training and coaching.

Functional fitness involves training for activities that we perform in our daily tasks, simulating the common movements that are performed at work, home or in sports. The functional exercises that have been included in Chapter 4 to develop your strength which makes it easier/safer to perform everyday activities without getting injured. An example of some of the activities that are simulated are: picking things up off the floor, putting things away over your head, carrying items, squatting down, reaching and rotating etc.

Each exercise focuses on more than one body part, instead of using one muscle e.g. the bicep curl, all of the muscles work together to produce more compound movements e.g. the bicep curl with a step up onto a box. This is an important concept in HIIT because all our muscles depend on each other and they also work together during daily activities. Thus, by using more compound movements during the training session; your daily movements will become more energy efficient by using less energy and reducing stress placed on the body.

Functional training works on different bodily movement planes, hitting different angles and building in the muscle stabilisers as well as using the main muscle groups. Many of the machines in the gym have pre-set angles and weights and don't allow complex movements that closely mirror everyday movements. However, some equipment such as the cables can be used and adapted to produce functional movements.

Some excellent equipment to use are kettlebells, Swiss Balls and/or body weight movements that mimic everyday activities. In addition, all of the compound exercises should engage the core; the core is essential to all basic movements within the body. This has the following positive impacts on your performance and health:

- Increases the body's ability to stabilize and generate from the core e.g. the deep abdominals, the hip rotators and the scapular stabilisers

- Improving the core is vital to good balance, stability and posture

- Increases the core strength due an increase in core stability

- Reduces   lower back, upper and lower extremity injuries

THE BENEFITS OF FUNCTIONAL TRAINING

HIIT resistance type exercises that only use one muscle are important for building muscle mass but unfortunately they can cause 'disproportion'. By adding functional exercises into your exercise routine, your balance, coordination and core stability will work together as a bodily unit, thereby enabling you to perform daily tasks a lot more efficiently[17]. This will lead to the following benefits:

- Makes daily tasks and activities a lot easier because the body is more conditioned

- Improves the overall musculoskeletal and joint function within the body

- Reduces the risk of injury and falling

- Enhances your quality of life

- Enhances stability, coordination and balance

- Develops strength in your muscle stabilizers e.g. shoulder, hip and core

- It boosts physical endurance

- Increases your resting metabolism because resting muscle requires more energy to function than fat

- Improves your posture by strengthening the lower back and core

- Helps to eliminate arthritic pain, back pain, upper extremity pain and joint pain e.g. the knee

- Improves range of motion at the joints e.g. the shoulder and hips.

References

(1) Talanian JL[6], Galloway SD[7], Heigenhauser GJ[8], Bonen A[9], Spriet LL[10].Two weeks of high-intensity aerobic interval training increases the capacity for fat oxidation during exercise in women.[11], J Appl Physiol. 2007])

(2) Stephen H. Boutcher, (2011) High-Intensity Intermittent Exercise and Fat Loss, Journal of Obesity, Volume 2011

(3) Tabata, I. (1996). Effects of moderate-intensity endurance and high-intensity intermittent training on anaerobic capacity and VO2max. Med Sci Sports Exerc.[12] 1996 Oct;28(10):1327-30.

(4) Wilmore J.H., Costill D.J. (2009) Physiology of Sport and Exercise. Human Kinetics, Champaign, Illinois.

(5) Rowan AE., Kueffner TE., Stavrianeas S., (2012). Short Duration High-Intensity Interval Training Improves Aerobic Conditioning of Female College Soccer Players. International Journal of Exercise Science. Jul2012, Vol. 5 Issue 3, p232-238.

(6) Helgerud J., Engen LC., Wisloff U., Hoff J., (2004) Aerobic endurance training improves soccer performance, Journal of Strength & Conditioning Research

(7) Dupont, Gregory, Akakpo, Koffi, Berthoin, Serge, (2010) The Effect of in-Season,High-Intensity Interval Training in Soccer Players, Journal of Strength & Conditioning Research

(8) T Gabbett, T King, D Jenkins,(2008). Applied physiology of rugby leagu[13]e Sports Medicine, 2008 February 2008, Volume 38, Issue 2[14], pp 119-138

(9) C Lorenzen, MD Williams, PS Turk, Paul S.; Meehan, Daniel L.; Kolsky, Daniel J. Cicioni,.(2000). Relationship Between Velocity Reached at VO 2max and Time-Trial

Performances in Elite Australian Rules Footballers.[15] International Journal of Sports Physiology & Performance .4 Issue 3, p408-411.

(10) Cregg, Cathal J (2013) Effects of high intensity interval training and high volume endurance training on maximal aerobic capacity, speed and power in club level gaelic football players. Master of Science thesis, Dublin City University.

(11) Santos E., Janeira M., Effects of Complex Training on Explosive Strength in Adolescent Male Basketball Players, Journal of Strength & Conditioning Research: May 2008 - Volume 22 - Issue 3 - pp 903-909[16])

(12) Talanian JL, et al. (2007).Two weeks of High-Intensity Aerobic Interval Training increases the capacity for fat oxidation during exercise in women. J Appl Physiol;102:1439-1447.

(13) Gibala, Martin J; Jonathan P. Little, Martin van Essen, Geoffrey P. Wilkin,(2006).Short-term sprint interval versus traditional endurance training: similar initial adaptations in human skeletal muscle and exercise performance". Journal of Physiology 575 (3): 901–911.

(14) Sharon A. Plowman, Denise L. Smith (2013). Exercise Physiology for Health Fitness and Performance. Wolters Kluwer Health

(15) Tanisho K, Hirakawa K.(2009).Training Effects on Endurance Capacity in Maximal Intermittent Exercise: Comparison Between Continuous and Interval Training. J Strength Cond Res. Oct 12.

(16) J. Helgerud, K. Høydal, E. Wang et al., "Aerobic high-intensity intervals improve VO2 max more than moderate training," Medicine and Science in Sports and Exercise, vol. 39, no. 4, pp. 665–671, 2007.

(17) William D. McArdle; Frank I. Katch; Victor L. Katch (2006). Essentials of exercise physiology[17]. Lippincott Williams & Wilkins. p.204. ISBN[18] 978-0-7817-4991-6[19].

(18) http://www.cdc.gov/nchs/nhanes.htm[20]

(19) Little JP, Gillen JB, Percival ME, Safdar A, Tarnopolsky MA, Punthakee Z, Jung ME, Gibala MJ. Low-volume high-intensity interval training reduces hyperglycemia and increases muscle mitochondrial capacity in patients with type 2 diabetes.[21] J Appl Physiol. 2011 Dec;111(6):1554-60.

(20) Helgerud et al. (2007). Aerobic high-intensity intervals improve VO2max more than moderate training. Med Sci Sports Exerc.[22] 2007 Apr;39(4):665-71

(21) Wisløff U[23], Nilsen TI[24], Drøyvold WB[25], Mørkved S[26], Slørdahl SA[27], Vatten LJ[28]. (2006). A single weekly bout of exercise may reduce cardiovascular mortality: how little pain for cardiac gain? 'The HUNT study, Norway'.Eur J Cardiovasc Prev Rehabil. 2Oct;13(5):798-804.

(22) Duncan S. Buchan1,*, Stewart Ollis1, John D. Young2, (2011). The effects of time and intensity of exercise on novel and established markers of CVD in adolescent youth; American Journal of Human Biology; Volume 23, Issue 4, pages 517–526.

(23) Min Lee & Ralph S. Paffenbarger, Jr. (200). Associations of Light, Moderate, and Vigorous Intensity Physical Activity with Longevity American Journal of Epidemiology Vol. 151, No. 3, p293-299.)

CHAPTER 3
THE SCIENCE BEHIND HIIT

This Chapter will focus on the mechanisms and the science that has been established through research in terms of HIIT. Some of the basic physiological systems will be explained briefly because this builds up the case for exercising with this very powerful and effective training method. We will endeavour not make this a science lesson in school, but add some scientific meat onto the bones and back it up with some robust and valid HIIT research. The following topics will be discussed:

- The science behind fat burning

- What really is the after burn effect?

- The 3 energy systems and how they relate to HIIT

- The fat burning hormones and HIIT

- The difference between genders and fat burning

- How HIIT can contribute to building muscle and strength

THE SCIENCE BEHIND FAT BURNING

The science behind fat burning becomes a whole lot easier to understand when you have a solid grasp of the changes that occur to the body post exercise. Some of the mechanisms are only activated with HIIT and not with any other form of conventional cardio.

The first phase of understanding the alterations brought on by HIIT is to determine the composition of skeletal muscle. Skeletal muscle is made up of 2 types of fibres and these are slow and fast twitch fibres. The ratio of the slow to fast twitch fibres is about 50:50[1] but these do vary slightly with genetics and your daily physical activity. The table below identifies the differences between the slow and fast twitch muscle fibres:

Slow Twitch Muscle Fibres	Fast Twitch Muscle Fibres
Contraction speed is slow	Contraction speed is fast
Contraction strength is low	Contraction strength is high
Fatigue resistance is high	Fatigue resistance is low
Aerobic capacity is high	Aerobic capacity is low
Anaerobic capacity is low	Anaerobic capacity is high
Myoglobin content is high	Myoglobin content is low
Mitochondria content is high	Mitochondria content is low
Capillary density is high	Capillary density is low

Source: Wilmore & Costill (2009)

From the table we can determine the major differences between slow and fast twitch muscle fibres. When slow twitch fibres contract the energy required is fundamentally produced by burning carbohydrates and fats with oxygen.

Slow twitch fibres can contract for longer periods of time than fast twitch fibres and recover almost immediately from the contraction. These are the endurance muscle fibres and work as long as they have a fuel source i.e. fats and carbs and when oxygen is present. These are the muscle fibres that are activated during low to moderate intensity bouts of activity.

On the other hand the fast twitch fibres are primarily activated during a bout of HIIT. From the table we can see that these types of muscle fibres contract very fast, with more force and take longer to recover after intense usage[2]. After a HIIT session your body can take up to 24 hours to repair and recover fully. This is well established as one of the main mechanisms for the increase in metabolism post exercise and this is needed for the body to recover/repair. This is backed up by the 2 following pieces of key research:

- Subjects who performed HIIT on an exercise cycle burned significantly more calories 24 hours post exercise than their counterparts who cycled at a moderate to steady state intensity[3].

- Another study discovered that subjects burnt 100 calories per day during the 24 hour window post exercise[4].

When we perform HIIT fast twitch fibres are activated and these have relatively poor oxygenation when compared to their slow twitch counterparts. Therefore, the fast twitch muscle fibres thrive in an anaerobic (without oxygen environment) and the anaerobic energy production is the major platform behind the benefits of HIIT. During explosive type exercises such as sprinting or weight lifting the energy is produced without the use of oxygen. Before we go any further a brief outline of the 3 main energy systems should be explained.

THE ENERGY SYSTEMS

1) The Phosphate Energy System (System 1)

This energy system consists of ATP (adenosine triphosphate) and CP (creatine phosphate). ATP is required in all muscle cells to be used as energy and without this vital source of energy the muscles can't contract. The CP is a short term energy system that is a catalyst for a very quick regeneration of ATP when the muscles contract. The phosphate system soon runs out and only lasts for a very short time. In fact think of this system as lasting for the first few seconds when you exercise!

2) The Aerobic System (System 2)

In the slow twitch muscle fibres the additional ATP is created by primarily burning carbohydrates and fats in the presence of oxygen. This continuous process occurs in the mitochondria within the muscle cells with the presence of oxygen. This production of ATP continues as long as oxygen and fuels are delivered to the muscle fibres.

In response to the increase in oxygen demand your heart rate also increases to pump the blood to the working muscles. This activity can be sustained to match the intensity of the exercise e.g. steady state cardio or until the fuel supply from the carbs and fats runs out. In the past it was this mechanism that was considered to be the best fat burner but this is now believed not to be the case. As we go through this Chapter you will understand why this approach is now believed to be out dated!

3) The Anaerobic Energy System (System 3)

During high intensity exercise the ATP/CP energy stores are used up very rapidly and your body struggles to deliver oxygen to the working muscles. Your heart rate and breathing rate does increase rapidly but despite this not enough oxygen is delivered to the fast twitch muscle fibres. As mentioned previously fast twitch fibres have a poor supply of oxygen, so while they initial use the aerobic system to create ATP, the lack of oxygen quickly forces the muscle cells to create energy without the means of oxygen.

The process is termed as 'anaerobic glycolysis' and this uses glucose as the primary fuel and not fat. The main by-product of the anaerobic energy system is lactic acid and this is produced at a very high rate. During a HIIT session the body very quickly uses up the ATP/CP and its glycogen stores and the hydrogen ions from the lactic acid build up quickly. These are the two main factors why the fast twitch muscles fatigue so quickly and this why you can only perform high intense bursts of activity for short periods of time e.g. sprinting.

THE ROLE OF HIIT ON THE 3 SYSTEMS AND ENERGY DEPLETION

Explosive HIIT training will help improve the ATP-CP pathway, thus improving explosive speed and power. This will help your body jump higher and sprint faster, but it WILL NOT increase your storage system for ATP-CP. This is why you will not be able to sustain a maximum intensity sprint for sustained periods of time. Remember anaerobic threshold means without oxygen, so it makes sense that your body is unable to sustain these maximum intensity bouts for much longer than 10 seconds. This is stage 1 of energy depletion during intense exercise.

STAGE 1

Stage 1 is not as challenging because you are using up your ATP and the short term CP energy stores. ATP is essential for contraction of the muscle fibers and CP is stored in your muscle cells and is converted to ATP very rapidly when ATP is needed. These two energy sources are used up within that first 10 seconds[5].

During less intense muscle contractions the ATP and CP energy systems are replenished by the aerobic energy system, which requires oxygen along with fats or carbohydrates as fuel.

During intense exercise like HIIT however, there just is not enough oxygen getting to your fast twitch muscle fibers for this to happen. This is another key difference between exercise that reaches anaerobic capacity and lesser intense forms of exercise that don't move past aerobic energy levels.

STAGE 2

With levels of ATP, CP and Oxygen running low we begin to enter Stage 2. This is the point of your HIIT workout that you will really have to reach past your comfort zone. You are now entering your lactic acid producing and anaerobic glycolysis stage.

If you recall we called this the 'anaerobic threshold'. By this time, your CP levels are running low, and anaerobic glycolysis will start to predominate.

As this stage continues, more and more lactic acid will begin to be produced. Lactic acid production is what signals this burning feeling in your muscles. If you have ever done highly intense workouts, you can attest to this feeling in your muscles.

When hydrogen ions accumulate in the muscles they cause the blood pH level to reach very low levels, temporary muscular fatigue results. Another limitation of the lactic acid system that relates to its anaerobic quality is that only a few moles of ATP can be resynthesized from the breakdown of sugar as compared to the yield possible when oxygen is present. This system can't be relied on for extended periods of time but is still vital during HIIT[2].

REDUCED FORCE PRODUCTION

CP levels can rapidly recover after exercise and return to 50 per cent of resting values in 1-2 minutes and to 90% of resting values after 3-4 minutes[2]. However, it can sometimes take up to 15 minutes for full re-synthesis in fast twitch fibres, which are depleted by the greatest extent during high intensity exercise such as HIIT training.

It is possible that glycogen depletion in fast twitch fibres may contribute to a reduced overall force production during a sprint. If an individual performs repeated sprints when muscle glycogen is depleted, fatigue often occurs earlier. Recovery of muscle glycogen, unlike CP or even pH can take over 24 hours to complete. Although the ability to deplete levels of CP increases the more anaerobically trained an individual is, there is evidence that those with a well-developed aerobic system can re-synthesise CP more rapidly than less trained individuals[5].

TRAINING EFFECT OF HIIT

As you do more HIIT sessions, you can increase the time it takes to reach this anaerobic threshold. In fact HIIT is actually an incredible way to increase your anaerobic threshold. After only a few weeks of HIIT you should already see an improvement. This means that you will be able to train at 100 percent intensity for longer periods of time. Your capacity for exercise and ability to burn fat will improve with consistent HIIT sessions[6].

When you are performing at 100 percent maximum intensity your oxygen levels begin to deplete as well. Your body tries to compensate by increasing your heart rate and breathing. This is why you are "out of breath" so to speak after running hard sprints. It is not physiologically possible to sprint at 100% for even a few minutes at a time since your ATP-CP levels are depleted and the lactic acid build up after a while would stop the muscles dead in their tracks. Anaerobic means without oxygen and it is only possible to train at maximum intensity in this state for a short duration of time.

HIIT requires a great deal of oxygen and lung capacity due to its very high intensity. When you are working at such a high intensity your anaerobic metabolism will predominate. Your body simply can't get oxygen to all of the places it needs it to go expeditiously. It is pushing your body to its limit, and using the less efficient anaerobic energy system to achieve maximal muscle power. This is one of the reasons that it is such an effective workout. In the case of HIIT – we are trading efficiency for intensity!

ANAEROBIC GLYCOLYSIS AND ACID ACCUMULATION

A quick recap- for very short, high intensity exercise (in the range of 1-10 seconds) the ATP/CP (system 1) is the predominant energy system that supplies most of the energy. For longer sprints there is a greater energy contribution from the anaerobic glycolysis system (system 3). The production of energy from the anaerobic glycolysis system takes about two seconds to reach its peak. However, after about 20 seconds of maximal exercise, the energy contribution from the anaerobic glycolysis system starts to decline due to many contributing factors such as 'acid accumulation'.

It was, until recently, commonly thought that lactic acid was a major cause of fatigue during high intensity and middle distance exercise. It has since been widely accepted that this is not the case as it is the hydrogen ions (H+) produced during glycolysis that is more likely to cause the fatigue[7]. In fact, lactate has been shown only to have beneficial effects as it actually decreases the level of hydrogen ions in the muscle and can also be converted to make glucose for the purpose of energy production.

One of the reasons that lactic acid is commonly measured by scientists and coaches is that it gives an indication of the changes in metabolism and acid levels, and can be used to monitor and set training programmes[8].

Due to the nature of HIIT being very explosive at a high 100% intensity a great deal of power will come from the anaerobic system but 'not all'! Energy is readily available during the anaerobic system but the pathways are not very efficient, with the energy stores often being depleted quickly, and a high level of lactic acid being produced as a by-product. HIIT is superb at producing lactic acid and some research from the California State University[9] concluded that lactic acid actually helps you to burn fat via the following mechanisms:

- It metabolises carbs quicker without increasing insulin levels or stimulating fat synthesis

- This enables more calories to be burned via an increase in carbs turn over without the adverse effect of spiked insulin levels (insulin will try to store carbs as fat)

- The body has to deal with high levels of lactic acid post exercise by using additional calories to lower the muscle pH back to normal levels

- High levels of lactic acid can trigger the release of human growth hormones (ref).

THE ROLE OF PHOSPHOFRUCTOKINASE (PFK)

One of the key enzymes (proteins that can speed up chemical reactions) involved in glycolysis is called phosphofructokinase (PFK) and is the main limiting factor in glycolysis. PFK activity can be enhanced as a result of anaerobic endurance training.

When lactic acid is produced during glycolysis, both in the muscle and the blood, buffering can take place. This is to prevent the build-up of acid by using buffers in the body such as bicarbonate.

Acid accumulation can cause fatigue as a result of mechanisms such as inhibition of enzymes involved in anaerobic glycolysis (PFK), interference with calcium binding and familiar pain or 'burn' felt when performing extended bouts of high intensity exercise[10].

One of the terms often associated with the anaerobic system, even though it is related to the aerobic system as well, is that it of excess Post-Exercise Oxygen Consumption (EPOC)[2].

WHAT IS THE AFTER BURN EFFECT?

Probably the biggest benefit of HIIT is the amount of calories you burn AFTER exercising.

EPOC is described as the 'amount of oxygen above resting requirements for a period of time after exercise has finished' and is similarly termed the after burn. It normally occurs following a demanding activity and eliminates the 'oxygen debt' within the body. EPOC is the process of returning the body back to its resting state by the use of oxygen and to counteract the metabolic actions that have occurred whilst performing HIIT[10].

When you burn glucose and glycogen without oxygen you are said to have reached your anaerobic threshold. By burning these fuels in the absence of oxygen your fast twitch muscle fibres overcome this limited delivery of oxygen.

During a HIIT session the fast twitch fibres predominately burn glucose as their primary fuel. A steady state cardio session predominately uses the slow twitch muscle fibres which use both fats and glucose as fuel.

Research has indicated that you do burn as many calories in both the HIIT and steady state cardio session but here comes the kicker; with HIIT you burn a vast amount more calories post exercise. This is called the 'after burn effect', or 'Post Exercise Oxygen Consumption', (EPOC) and this probably the biggest benefit of performing HIIT- the amount of calories that are burnt after you stop exercising[11].

After you stop your steady state cardio your slow twitch muscle fibres recover very quickly. This actually means the slow twitch muscle fibres have repaired any moderate damage and the ATP levels within these fibres are replenished to their pre-exercise levels. It is due to the fact that the slow twitch fibres actually recover so quickly that it hinders *all* of the metabolic benefits from the exercise session.

This is where HIIT blasts steady state cardio out of the water in terms of its fat burning potential. Bear in mind that it can take up to 24 hours for the fast twitch muscle fibres to repair themselves fully after a HIIT[10] session . Due to the intensity of the exercises and the increased recruitment of the fast twitch fibres during the session; this is considered to the major reasons why the body takes so long to repair itself.

Your body post exercise after a HIIT session is working very hard to repair the fast twitch muscle fibres and to replenish the ATP stocks. This process raises your metabolism to cope with the demand of the repairing and replenishing process and this equates to an increase in calories burnt!

Research has indicated that this increase in calories burned can last up to 24 hours after a HIIT session [11]. When you perform HIIT three times per week in essence your resting metabolism will be rocketed up by an additional 72 hours per week (12 &13). HIIT definitely speeds up your fat burning potential and your weight loss goals are achieved far quicker than performing conventional boring cardio.

Performing HIIT 3 times per week equates to the same calorie burning output as performing conventional cardio 6 times per week. Theoretically you are exercising for 3 days but have an additional 3 days of fat burning with HIIT. Research has shown an improvement in the following metabolic markers post exercise[14].

- An increase in Glut-4 content in the muscle and glucose transport activity

- An improved fatty acid oxidative enzyme in the skeletal muscle and this improves fat metabolism

THE DURATION OF EPOC

The effect of EPOC is at its highest point straight after the cessation of your HIIT session and it tapers off gradually. One study noted that EPOC reduced to around 13% three hours post exercise and dropped to 4% around the 16 hour mark post exercise[15].

Another piece of research discovered that HIIT's after burn effect was still evident around the 38 hour mark post exercise!

THE MAGNITUDE OF THE EPOC EFFECT

There is evidence to suggest that EPOC is present after both aerobic and anaerobic exercise(15 & 16). Regardless of the difference in some experimental design there are indeed similar outcomes from the investigations and these are simplified as follows:

- Anaerobic exercise burns more calories post exercise but there is a similar amount of calories burnt in both regimes (aerobic versus anaerobic)

- HIIT increases the amount of subcutaneous fat burnt even though fewer calories were burnt during the actual session

- If the work output is the same during both an anaerobic and aerobic session, the EPOC is still greater after the anaerobic session

- EPOC increases significantly with the intensity of the exercise. Therefore you burn more calories after a HIIT session than a conventional cardio session.

WHY YOUR BODY GOES INTO EPOC AFTER A HIIT SESSION

When your body enters into EPOC after a HIIT session it can cause you to enter into a state of severe 'oxygen debt'. This oxygen debt has to be repaid somehow and it this process that enables the body to go back to a state of equilibrium.

However, you may be thinking why does my body actually enter into a state of EPOC after a HIIT session? There is a vast amount of research out there and this section will briefly summarise the main reasons why your body goes into EPOC. A key point to remember is that a large amount of oxygen, fuel and energy is needed during EPOC to restore the body back to a state of equilibrium; the main mechanisms that need restoring are as follows(15 &16):

- High levels of circulating fat burning hormones, which need balancing out
- To replenish stored glycogen levels in the muscle and liver needed for energy
- ATP and creatine phosphate levels need to be restored
- Muscle cell damage needs to be repaired
- High levels of hormones and signalling compounds within the nervous system need balancing and restoring
- Your muscle pH needs restoring from an acidic state
- An increase in body temperature caused by all of these metabolic reactions needs to be lowered back down to the normal level.

GENDER DIFFERENCES IN FAT METABOLISM

It is well established that women tend to have a higher % body fat than men. Men and women also differ where their body fat is stored. Hormones, hormone receptors and enzymes all play a contributing role towards fat metabolism.

Before we go on to discuss the different types of hormones, lets us firstly discuss how fat is metabolized in both genders.

THE DIFFERENCE BETWEEN FAT METABOLISM AND FAT MOBILISATION

'Fat mobilisation' is a process of releasing fats from storage sites within the body and 'fat metabolism' is the method of how the body breaks down the fats so that they can be used as a fuel source. Hormone sensitive lipase (HSL) and lipoprotein lipase (LPL) are the two hormones that the body uses to regulate the *mobilization* of free fatty acids.

Hormone sensitive lipase is located within the actual fat cells and it releases fat due to the signalling of cyclic AMP (cyclic adenosine monophosphate is a second messenger that is used for intracellular signalling, and it helps to transfer hormones that couldn't pass through the cell membrane). This is impacted by the activity hormone receptors in the fat cells called the 'adrenergic receptors'(7&12). When HSL is secreted it helps to break down triglycerides in the adipose tissue into 3 free fatty acids (FFAs) and one glycerol. This mechanism of breaking down the triglycerides into fatty acids and glycerol is called 'lipolysis'.

When the free fatty acids are in the blood stream, they attach themselves to 'albumin' which is the main vehicle that the FFAs use to travel. Once the free fatty acids arrive at the muscle cells, they are transported into the cells via the following 3 transporters:

- Fatty acid binding proteins
- Fatty acid translocase
- Fatty acid transport proteins

The 3 protein transporters then carry the FFA's across the muscle cell's membrane and into the mitochondria to be oxidised. The additional glycerol molecule that is created during lipolysis is either oxidised in the liver and/or used in the breakdown of glucose and/or to create more triglycerides.

THE ROLE OF LIPOPROTEIN LIPASE

Lipoprotein lipase is located in the blood vessel walls of the circulatory system, in adipose tissue and within the liver. Fundamentally, lipoprotein lipase acts upon the triglycerides within the lipoproteins in the blood, and these lipoproteins are vehicles that carry cholesterol and triglycerides for fat storage. Triglycerides are then broken down into free fatty acids and used as fuel or stored in the liver as resynthesized triglycerides. Lipoprotein lipase controls the amount of fat that is stored in sites around the body[12].

THE MAJOR ROLE OF THE CATECHOLAMINES AND FAT BURNING

There is evidence to suggest that HIIT actually boosts your catecholamine levels[17]. The catecholamines are the primary catalyst for lipolysis. They bind to the adipocytes and muscle cells, and can either block or the activate hormone sensitive lipase. Catecholamines have 2 main types of receptors and often these receptors can be found in the same cells:

1. Alpha receptors-these *inhibit* lipolysis (A = anti burn) and they decrease blood flow to a specific area.

2. Beta receptors- these help to *active* lipolysis (B= burn) and they increase blood flow to a specific area.

However, the receptor available and its sensitivity or resistance of the catecholamines will determine the overall response of hormone sensitive lipase within the cells. In addition, the higher the amount of alpha or beta receptors within the cells will determine the response of the hormone sensitive lipase. For example, abdominal adipocytes are more sensitive to beta receptor stimulation by the catecholamines compared to the hip/thigh in both genders. Therefore, abdominal fat is easier to mobilise than hip/thigh fat in women, as they have an increased number of alpha receptors in the thigh/hip area.

This is the main rationale why women tend to store fat in the fat/thigh area (pre-menopausal); combined with differences in the type and number of fat cells in the lower body region[8]. Hence, this could be a leading factor in the fat distribution differences between both sexes.

Another mechanism associated with fat distribution differences between both genders is the amount of lipoprotein lipase in various cells. Women tend to increased levels of lipoprotein lipase within the hip/thigh area in comparison to the abdominal region. In addition, women's lower body subcutaneous fat has a higher amount of estrogen receptors which makes it very stubborn to burn.

Wilmore and Costill (2009) postulated that women have 10 times more alpha receptor cells than men, and the hormone oestrogen increases the number and activity of the alpha receptor cells. In addition, a female's subcutaneous fat has more alpha cells when compared to males, and this maybe a key rational why it's difficult to shift the fat in the hip, thigh regions and lower belly regions for women compared to men.

However, men do have a higher saturation of alpha cells in the belly area compared to women.

However, it is *not always* this cut and dry because hormones not only inform the body how to use the fuel but behave differently depending on their ratios with other hormones. A good example of this is the ratio of insulin to catecholamines which are a major factor in fat storage. In addition if insulin and the catecholamines are both high, fat storage is reduced. On the other hand, if the raise in insulin is unopposed by the catecholamines, fat storage is increased because insulin increases LPL activity and suppresses HSL activity. Insulin impairs the normal function of beta receptors, which is another form of blocking HSL.

THE RELATIONSHIP BETWEEN INSULIN AND THE CATECHOLAMINES

With the fat burning potential of the catecholamines being absent, the fat storage of insulin is increased. In addition, the catecholamines can speed up fat release when they bind to the beta receptors which would increase the HSL activity. On the other hand, they can slow down fat metabolism when they combine with the alpha receptors. This one of the main reasons that stubborn fat, which has a higher number of alpha receptors, is harder to shift.

Another key point to remember is that the alpha receptors reduce blood flow to the areas that are holding onto the subcutaneous fat; which reduces the body's fat mobilisation potential[7].

WHAT IS GLUT4?

GLUT4 is an important hormone transporter which is boosted by HIIT[18]. GLUT4 is found in muscle and adipose tissue; it is transported to plasma membrane as a result of the increased levels of insulin. This helps to move the glucose into the cells ready to be broken down and used as a prime energy source. However, prolonged levels of insulin and cortisol inhibit GLUT4 gene transcription and this can result in the reduction of glucose entering into the muscle. Subsequently, the blood glucose in the body is then stored as fat; which is not very good news for you.

LET'S NOT FORGET ABOUT TESTOSTERONE

HIIT can trigger an increase in testosterone levels because you are exercising at a 100% V02 max intensity [19]. Testosterone is anabolic hormone that builds muscle and increase your body's fat burning potential. How does testosterone burn fat?

Well, the fat cells are richly saturated with androgen receptors and adipose tissue is the key target for testosterone. One of the main roles of testosterone is to augment the density of the beta receptors and as mentioned previously they are controlled by the catecholamines. Therefore, if testosterone binds to the adipose cells it will indirectly burn the fat. If the beta receptors are boosted it takes less catecholamines to burn the fat via lipolysis.

In biochemical terms, the androstenedione enhances fat sensitivity during lipolysis and some of the androstenedione in the bloodstream is converted into testosterone within the adipose tissue. The sensitising make up of testosterone is backed up by the presence of the growth hormone. There is a very clear pathway and relationship between the catecholamines and HGH in up-regulating the beta receptors. Testosterone can be a catalyst for the release of HGH [7], and both hormones have the same metabolic reactions in creating muscle anabolism. Also testosterone can block fat uptake in the adipose cells, and this mechanism can stop fat storage -

the catecholamines can not only prevent fat release but also block the fat from entering the cells.

The mitochondria in the cells have testosterone binding sites and these increase the speed at which the fat enters the cells. Again this is controlled by the catecholamines and the rate of entry will determine the amount of fat that is burnt. The higher the rate of entry into the mitochondria; the higher its fat burning potential! The enhanced rate of fat oxidation caused by the catecholamines is very useful for weight loss!

THE ROLE OF THE MITOCHONDRIA

A quick reminder is that the mitochondria are the energy factory of the human cells and this is where ATP is generated as a result of burning fats and carbs in the presence of oxygen. HIIT increases the number and size of the mitochondria in the slow twitch fibres (mitochondrial density)[20] and this increases the muscle's ability to burn fat. On the other hand there is evidence to suggest that lengthy conventional steady state cardio actually damages the structure of the mitochondria and reduces your fat burning potential.

The increase in mitochondrial density ensures that more energy (ATP) is available to the working muscles and this produces a greater force for a longer duration. HIIT can cause physiological changes that mirror the results of endurance training but actually different signalling pathways are being activated to achieve similar results in a shorter period of time. Hence, high volume training activates the CaMK (signaling pathway in fast-to-slow fiber type transformation) pathway and HIIT activates the AMPK (master regulator of cellular energy) pathway! Either way an increase in the levels of the mitochondria in the slow twitch muscle fibres improves your muscle's capacity for oxygen consumption and improved athletic endurance!

THE MUSCULAR SYSTEM AND HIIT

WHAT IS MUSCULAR ENDURANCE?

Using moderate weight with higher reps and lower rest intervals will drastically improve your 'muscular endurance'. Muscular endurance is the body's ability to create and maintain force production for prolonged periods of time. This helps to build joint stability, core strength and it's the foundation of your body's strength and power whilst running. Research has indicated that strength training programs using high reps with moderate weight are the best protocols for boosting your muscular endurance levels. On the other hand, resistance training protocols that use low to moderate repetition ranges with a progressive overload can lead to muscle hypertrophy[2].

WHAT IS MUSCULAR STRENGTH?

Strength is defined as 'the ability of the body to produce any internal force to overcome any external force'. The internal force produced within the muscles is what facilitates force production and low repetition with heavy weight does initially increase the neuromuscular system. However, traditional strength training solely focuses on developing maximal strength in individual muscle groups, within one plane of motion and with a heavy weight/low rep range. This isolated muscle group approach when strength training is not the best option for runners. Using heavy weights does increase the number of motor units recruited and the neural demand of muscle fibres, especially in the early stages of resistance training.

However, here comes the kicker, even when using heavier weights there is a plateau in strength and any further increases in strength have been attributed to muscle hypertrophy. A good strength program does not want to induce a rapid plateau in strength or hypertrophy but should focus on stabilizing your body's movement system and muscular endurance, which are important platforms for improving your strength.

THE IMPACT OF HIIT

HIIT activates and increases the size of the fast twitch muscle fibres and it is this process that has been linked to increases in strength[21]. This goes hand in hand with the impact that HIIT has on building and maintaining lean muscle mass via some key hormonal changes.

As mentioned previously, HIIT has been shown to have positive effects on human growth hormone (HGH) levels which are very important for building muscle, especially when combined with the right resistance program. This combination of HIIT and resistance training ensures that your body is both a fat burning and muscle building machine.

For optimal fat burning and growth hormone release the best work out programs should consist of high reps with moderate weight until failure; then have a short rest interval in between the next set[8]. This type of training will increase the amount of lactic acid produced, and there is a close connection between high lactic acid levels and the increased amount of HGG that are available.

Increasing your HGH levels will have a dramatic effect on boosting your lean muscle mass and the body's fat burning potential. Naturally increasing your HGH levels is one of the best methods of maximizing your composition goals, preserving and building lean body mass. Moderate conventional cardio does not trigger the release of HGH because it does not cause a build-up of lactic acid. Again the high intensity nature of the HIIT exercise session is the main catalyst for increased HGH and lactic acid production. HGH is essential for muscle growth and development but it also has the following roles within the body(7&8):

- It is the major hormone that is involved in the growth and development of children and adolescents e.g. it plays a key role in the height of a human

- It stimulates the grow of the major organs e.g. the brain

- It increases calcium retention which strengthens and increases the mineralisation of bone

- It helps to maintain a balanced metabolic status within the body

- It increases protein synthesis for the development of muscle tissue

- It promotes glucose production in the liver

- It contributes to the function of the pancreatic islets and these are essential for the production of insulin

- It stimulates immune function

There is evidence to suggest that that HGH levels are inflated to around 500 times of their resting values after a HIIT session is completed at a maximum intensity(22&23). In addition, exercising your fast twitch muscles at their peak capacity is proven to boost HGH, burn fat and to build muscle tissue.

The main beneficial mechanism associated with building muscle is the increase in protein synthesis to create muscle tissue. It is a double positive because HIIT causes maximum stress and micro tears within the skeletal muscle, by shocking them. This mechanism activates the recovery process within the skeletal tissue and this is the 'basic' catalyst for muscle growth, by recruiting reserve or stubborn muscle fibres. This shock to the muscle created by the increased stress caused by HIIT induces hypertrophy and muscle growth. The muscle growth is further boosted by the impact of the HGH on the creation of muscle tissue!

HIIT CAN LIMIT MUSCLE LOSS DURING CARDIO

HIIT is a very popular form of cardio training for body builders and fitness athletes because your body will not lose any muscle mass during training. In fact – HIIT can actually help you with your lean muscle gains. As mentioned previously HIIT raises your HGH levels and for the human body this is the hormone responsible for muscle growth. Raising your HGH levels naturally is a very important factor that maximizes your body's potential to gain lean muscle mass.

Since HIIT trains your fast twitch muscle fibers, it is incredibly beneficial for strength, power, and lean muscle mass. Your fast twitch muscle fibers are great for any kind of explosive movement, and training them, with HIIT, can help you in the weight room since you are using the same muscle fibers with resistance training.

The shorter cardio workouts and fast twitch muscle utilization make HIIT the perfect storm for any body builder or physique athlete concerned with losing muscle mass during cardio. It has been proven that long static cardio sessions are horrible for preserving and building lean muscle. This is because long distance and static cardio decreases your testosterone(T), and creates a major calorie deficit. A study by the University of British Columbia[29] found that male runners who pounded over 40 miles of pavement per week had distinctly lower T levels than their short-distance running counterparts[24].

Long distance cardio will put you at a major calorie deficit as well. Remember that HIIT targets fat, but moderate cardio will cause you to lose weight - both fat and muscle. When trying to preserve lean muscle mass stick with HIIT as it has been shown to have anabolic effects on your body much better than standard cardio. Any kind of aerobic training done for long periods of time will have adverse effects to your strength training since this is predominantly a slow twitch muscle exercise.

With HIIT you truly are getting the best of both worlds. It will not mess up your strength pathways and protein synthesis, which could have catabolic effects.

USING COMPOUND EXERCISES AND HIIT

Compound exercises are movements that are multi-jointed in nature and they use several muscle groups to help to move your limbs. They can improve joint stability, overall balance, co-ordination and reaction time. They closely resemble functional exercises and include the following:

- Squats
- Deadlifts
- Lunges
- Rows
- Presses

When executing these compound exercises you will be recruiting more muscle fibres and this translates to building a solid foundation in body strength, and in time enhanced overall strength gains. They also increase the energy expended during the work outs and help to burn fat up to 24 hours post exercise[7]. This boost in total energy turn-over has been predominantly attributed to the increase in muscle fibre recruitment and the actual energy required powering the skeletal muscle. The net result is an increase in overall calorie expenditure and improved weight maintenance.

On the other hand isolated exercise such as the bicep curl and tricep extensions are a waste of time because they recruit smaller amounts of muscle groups. They are used for shaping the muscle in bodybuilding and they have a lack of cardiovascular effect, very limited strength gains and fat burning potential with *no* after burn effect. They are best left alone unless you are recovering from certain types of small muscle group injuries.

References

(1) Ingalls C.P. (2004) Nature vs. nurture: can exercise really alter fiber type composition in human skeletal muscle? Journal of Applied Physiology November 1, 2004 vol. 97 no. 5 1591-1592.[30]

(2) Wilmore. J.H, Costill D,J (2009)Physiology of Sport and Exercise. Human Kinetics. Champaign, Illinois.

(3) Treuth MS, Hunter GR, Williams M. (1996) Effects of exercise intensity on 24-h energy expenditure and substrate oxidation. Med Sci Sports Exerc. Sep;28(9):1138-43.

(4) Jeffrey Warren King, (2001) A Comparison of the Effects of Interval Training vs. Continuous Training on Weight Loss and Body Composition in Obese Pre-Menopausal Women. Electronic Theses and Dissertations, East Tennessee State University

(5) Powers S. Howley J (2011) - Exercise Physiology: Theory and Application to Fitness and Performance. McGraw-Hill Education

(6) J. Laforgia[31]a, R. T. Withers[32]b & C. J. Gore[33]c (1997). Effects of exercise intensity and duration on the excess post-exercise oxygen consumption, Journal of Sports Sciences, pages 1247-1264

(7) William D. McArdle; Frank I. Katch; Victor L. Katch (2006). Essentials of exercise physiology[34]. Lippincott Williams & Wilkins. p. 204. ISBN[35] 978-0-7817-4991-6[36].

(8) Sharon A. Plowman, Denise L. Smith (2013). Exercise Physiology for Health Fitness and Performance. Wolters Kluwer Health

(9) http://fitnessblackbook.com/interval-training/how-interval-training-works-lactic-acid-oxygen-debt-and-recovery/

(10) Talanian, Jason L.; Stuart D. R. Galloway, George J. F. Heigenhauser, Arend Bonen, Lawrence L. Spriet (2007). "Two weeks of high-intensity aerobic interval training increases the capacity for fat oxidation during exercise in women". Journal of Applied Physiology[37] 102 (4): 1439-1447.

(11) Perry, Christopher G.R.; Heigenhauser, George J.F.; Bonen, Arend; Spriet, Lawrence L. (2008). "High-intensity aerobic interval training increases fat and carbohydrate metabolic capacities in human skeletal muscle"[38]. Applied Physiology, Nutrition, and Metabolism[39] 33 (6): 1112-1123.

(12) King, Jeffrey W.. A Comparison of the Effects of Interval Training vs. Continuous Training on Weight Loss and Body Composition in Obese Pre-Menopausal Women (M.A. thesis). East Tennessee State University.

(13) Elisabet Børsheim, Roald Bahr, Effect of Exercise Intensity, Duration and Mode on Post-Exercise Oxygen Consumption, Sports Medicine, December 2003, Volume 33, Issue 14, pp 1037-1060

(14) Borsheim E., Bahr R. Effect of Exercise Intensity, Duration and Mode on Post-Exercise Oxygen Consumption, Sports Medicine, December 2003, Volume 33, Issue 14, pp 1037-1060

(15) Schuenke MD, Mikat RP, McBride JM (2002). "Effect of an acute period of resistance exercise on excess post-exercise oxygen consumption: implications for body mass management". European Journal of Applied Physiology 86 (5): 411–7

(16) Bahr R (1992). "Excess postexercise oxygen consumption--magnitude, mechanisms and practical implications". Acta Physiologica Scandinavica. Supplementum 605: 1–70

(17) Bahr R, Høstmark AT, Newsholme EA, Grønnerød O, Sejersted OM (1991). "Effect of exercise on recovery changes in plasma levels of FFA, glycerol, glucose and catecholamines". Acta Physiologica Scandinavica 143 (1): 105–15.

(18) Terada S, Yokozeki T, Kawanaka K, Ogawa K, Higuchi M, Ezaki O, Tabata I. Effects of high-intensity swimming training on GLUT4 and glucose transport activity in rat skeletal muscle. J Appl Physiol. 90_(6): 2019-2024, 2001

(19) http://www.muscleandperformancemag.com/training/2012/7/power-hiit[40]

(20) Daussin FN., Zoll J., Dufour SP., Ponsot E., Lonsdorfer-Wolf., Doutreleau S., Mettauer B., Piquard F., Geny B. and Richard R.Effect of interval versus continuous training on cardiorespiratory and mitochondrial functions: relationship to aerobic performance improvements in sedentary subjects, Am J Physiol Regul Integr Comp Physiol, April 2008, 295:R264-R272, 2008.

(21) Fitts R.H., Widrick J.J.(1996) Muscle mechanics: adaptations with exercise-training. Exercise and Sport Sciences Reviews , 24:427-473[41]

(22) S. E. Gordon[42], W. J. Kraemer[43], N. H. Vos[44], J. M. Lynch[45], and H. G. Knuttgen[46], Effect of acid-base balance on the growth hormone response to acute high-intensity cycle exercise, Journal of Applied Physiology February 1, 1994 vol. 76 no. 2 821-829

(23) Luger A. · Watschinger B. · Deuster P. · Svoboda T. · Clodi M. · Chrousos G.P., Plasma Growth Hormone and Prolactin Responses to Graded Levels of Acute Exercise and to a Lactate Infusion, Neuroendocrinology 1992;56:112-117)

(24) http://testosteroneandyou.com/

CHAPTER 4
THE WORK OUTS

This Chapter is where the hard work begins and all of the information is pulled together from the previous sections of the book, so that you can have all of the benefits of HIIT. The primary focus of this Chapter is for you to perform the 10 HIIT work outs over an 8 week period, so that you achieve your goal of losing some body weight. It will help you along the way by showing you how to set goals, how to track them by using apps and some top training advice to keep you on target with your goals.

As mentioned previously, all of the work-outs can be performed at home or in the gym and they cater for all fitness levels. To ascertain your fitness level a fitness test has been incorporated, this will determine what work outs you should be performing.

All of the warm up, cool down, foam roller and exercises within the 10 work outs have been fully explained in the 'exercise descriptions' part of the Chapter. So lace up those training shoes and let's get going!

TRAINING GOALS

Goal setting is very important when on your weight loss and fitness journey. It is also an easy method to keeping you on track throughout the 8 weeks. Each of the goals can be adjusted to suit your needs. This will ensure that the program is sustainable and successful!

The SMART approach is a very simple to use goal setting model and it really does work. Try to keep the goals basic and follow the framework below, in addition there is an example for you to follow!

A basic example of some SMART weight loss goals:

- **Specific** - To lose 8 kgs or 17 pounds in 8 weeks
- **Measurable** - measure success of training plans by using training diaries
- **Adjustable** - adjust any of the goals to achieve the weekly / 8 weeks outcomes.
- **Realistic** - fitting training in with work and home schedule
- **Time** - 8 weeks

Now take 10 minutes to write down your training goals:

- Specific -
- Measurable -
- Adjustable -
- Realistic -
- Time -

USING A TRAINING DIARY

A dairy is an important part of training, it can be used to monitor and track your progress whilst using the training plans. Record any successes that you have in terms of the HIIT approach and note exercises that you discovered to be too difficult or easy. As you go through the 8 week plan you will find that the exercises do start to become a lot easier because your body has adapted to them.

You can track your work outs by using phone apps, as they are a great resource and usually free! *Map my Fitness*, *Fitnessstar* and *Fitness Fast* are some examples of good quality phone apps. However feel free to do your own research and find an app that suits your training needs.

TRAINING TIPS TO KEEP YOU ON TRACK

- If possible exercise with a buddy; this definitely helps with your training goals. The right partner can give you a push when you need it and vice versa.

- Stick to the training plans, as this shows commitment and determination. They have been specifically designed to maximise weight loss and increase your fitness levels.

- You will have to train on Saturdays; don't cheat and think that you can double up the next day. This throws the training plan out of sync and keeping on track is important.

- Get into a routine, pack your kit bag by the front door and have your trainers next to the bed. This is a very important motivational tool!

- Rest days are important for your physical and mental recovery, stay focused and on track even on these days and try to use the foam roller.

- Record notes in your training diary and look at how much you have improved.

- Give 100% effort to every training session and remember that 8 weeks will soon fly by.

- If you get injured or experience any side effects, have some time out and see a doctor or physiotherapist. You will heal quicker.

- Keep hydrated when working out and give the booze a miss or modify your intake - especially on rest days!

- Be positive and focus on that finishing line/ physique goals in 8 weeks

- Remember there are no short cuts!!

- The correct footwear is important, if you can afford to buy trainers that are measured to your feet. The right footwear will prevent injuries and keep up on track.

- Last by no means least....ENJOY!!!

THE TRAINING PLANS

We are finally here- this is where the hard work really kicks in!

The 10 work out plans have been differentiated in terms of fitness ability i.e. beginner, intermediate and advanced. There is a self- assessment fitness test that will establish your fitness level, from which you will be able to determine what level of the work outs you should be using e.g. beginner versus intermediate. In addition, it has an accompanying warm up and cool-down routine that you should use with each of the 10 work outs.

If you have not exercised for a while, don't worry as each work out has been designed to get you moving in a comfortable but challenging way. This is the advantage of HIIT training because it is a lot short and sharper with maximum weight loss results. You will start to feel and look different, and use this positive momentum to drive your fitness levels up!

You will initially lose a lot of weight when using the training plans when combined with the diet advice in Chapter 5. A healthy weight loss is 2-3 pounds per week and this is a very healthy range. If you crash the weight off then you are more likely to put it back on- with interest! The more gradual your weight loss, the less likely that is will not return and this is by far the best strategy to follow!

SELF-ASSESSMENT FITNESS TEST

The first step is for you to assess your fitness levels and this will indicate what work out level you should be following i.e. beginner, intermediate or advanced. The test is very easy to use, so just read the instructions and practice the test. When you are confident perform the test, record your results and compare against the fitness classification table (following page).

INSTRUCTIONS

This test is designed to measure cardio vascular fitness, and can be completed at home very easily in 4 minutes. Cardio vascular fitness is how effective the heart and its associated vessels are at pumping your blood around the body when exercising or at rest. The '8 week program overview' (following page) is connected to your baseline fitness levels, so just follow this and wave goodbye to your body fat!

Please follow these simple testing guidelines:

Exercise:

Using the lower step on the stairs in your home; step up and down for three minutes. Step up with one foot and then the other; contact the step with the entire sole of the foot plus the heel.

Method

1. Then step down with one foot followed by the other foot, allow the heel to contact the floor as this aids whole body absorption. Also keep the body weight on the foot which is still in contact with the step.

2. Try to maintain a steady four beat rhythm, which should consist of two 'ups' and two 'downs'. Visualise this rhythm in your head.

3. Use your arms as stabilisers for better balance, and with a marching action; pump them alternatively to the legs.

4. At the end of the 3 minutes, stay standing and take your wrist pulse for 1 minute. Then compare your results to the fitness classification chart below.

Safety Points

- Check that the step on the stairs is not polished wood or has loose carpet, as this will be too slippery to complete the test.

- The height of the step should not cause the knee joint to flex to 90 degrees or more when fully loaded. If it does flex to 90 degrees or over, then the step too high and you may have to find an alternative platform.

- Try to step softly as this avoids high impact

- Look at the step periodically for improved foot placement and make heel contact every time, and always keep your toes and knees facing forward.

- Don't over extend the back or knees anytime; and when stepping up lean from the ankles and not the waist. Remember that if you over extend the natural curve of the spine this is when injuries start to occur.

- You can practice a couple of times until you get the hang of the test

The Correct Technique for Taking the Pulse at the Wrist

- Remain standing and don't sit down, as this will give an inaccurate measurement.

- Never use your thumb as this has its own pulse.

- Place the second and third fingers on the crease of the wrist which is below the base of the thumb

- Press lightly until you find a pulse or move both fingers until you feel the pulse.

- Hold your arm down towards the floor

- Begin timing for 60 seconds once you have found it.

- Practice this technique a few times, as this is important in getting an accurate heart measurement straight after the 3 minute test. If you can't find the pulse at your wrist, then try to find it in your neck.

The next step is to use the fitness classification table below and to calculate what is your fitness level. It really is as simple as that!

3 Minute Step Test, Pulse Rate (beats per minute) and Fitness Classifications Table

Work Out Level	Age	18-25	26-35	36-45	46-55	56-65	65+
Advanced	Excellent	<85	<88	<90	<94	<95	<90
Advanced	Good	85-98	88-99	90-102	94-104	95-104	90-102
Intermediate	Above Average	99-108	100-111	103-110	105-115	105-112	103-115
Intermediate	Average	109-117	112-119	111-118	116-120	113-118	116-122
Beginner	Below Average	118-126	120-126	119-128	121-129	119-128	123-128
Beginner	Poor	127-140	127-138	129-140	130-135	129-139	129-134
Beginner	Very Poor	>140	>138	>140	>135	>139	>134

Source: Canadian Public Health Association Project

8 WEEK PROGRAM OVERVIEW

The 8 week programs have been designed to improve your cardio fitness, upper body and lower body strength. In addition, our 'HIIT' (High Intensity Interval Training) style of training will ensure that pounding the pavements for hours on end is a thing of the past and that you are 'fighting fit' and that your fat is shredded forever!

The 10 work outs have been adapted, so that you can use them at home and/or at the gym. Some of the exercises you can perform in the gym and not at home because you may not have the equipment - not to worry as some have been altered to suit home use. This will be highlighted throughout the work outs and should keep you on track for your weight loss whether you are at home or at the gym!

Week Nos	Mon	Tues	Wed	Thurs	Frii	Sat
1 & 2	WO A	WO B	REST	WO C	WO D	WO E
3 & 4	WO A	WO B	REST	WO C	WO D	WO E
5 & 6	WO F	WO G	WO H	REST	WO I	WO J
7 & 8	WO F	WO G	WO H	REST	WO I	WO J
*KEY: WO = WORK OUT + LETTER OF WORK OUT e.g. WO A = WO1						
SUNDAY = REST						

Try to perform the work outs without missing a day of training, however if you do miss a day just keep following the plan and try to keep it in the same order. Try to commit to at least 3 days per week and you will see your body begin to change and the weight will start to drop off! The rest days have been placed in the program to help you to relax and to get you prepared for your next work out. So enjoy the 8 week program and start to see a new you.

NUMBER OF TIMES TO REPEAT WORK OUTS FOR EACH WEEK (PURPLE TABLE).

Week Number			
	Beginner	Intermediate	Advanced
1-4	2	3	4
5-8	3	4	5

All of the 10 works out have are based around a HIIT model i.e. 8 x 20-40 seconds of high intensity activity with 10-30 seconds rest intervals. As you get fitter you will be able to repeat the work outs more than once and the amount of times that you repeat the HIIT work outs during each session is shown in the *PURPLE Table* above.

All of the work outs are a mixture of compound movements where you use all of the large muscle groups and are a variety of high intensity cardio, bodyweight resistance and free weights all designed to burn stubborn fat. The work outs have been created to get maximum results in a short period of time and all you need is commitment, dedication and some free time set a-side.

EQUIPMENT

The equipment has been split into essential and optional (to buy) for the home work outs. You can borrow all of the equipment at the gym, if you are a member of course. Splitting the equipment into essential and optional increases the accessibility and valuable factor of the work outs. Everyone can perform the home works outs; all you need is some dumbbells, a Swiss ball and a chair.

Essential for Home Use	Optional /Gym Use
Swiss Ball	Barbell*
Chair	
Dumbbells*	
Foam Roller	

*see Weights below for weight

SOME TOP TIPS

A top tip is to look at the next day's work out plan and determine what equipment is required. Before the session, some good practice is to set up the equipment in your work space, so that you can move to it during the 10-30 second rest intervals. In addition, always prepare water before the work outs, as you will need to take lots on board.

WEIGHTS (Please use this advice with all of the Dumbbell/Barbell Exercises)

A good starting point for using the dumbbell/barbell weight is 4 kgs for a woman and 7 kgs for a man. You can increase or decrease accordingly throughout the program and remember that the weight used should be comfortable to lift but challenging. If you don't own any dumbbells then use water bottles and weigh the bottle when adding the water.

In terms of using the weights, try to pump out as many reps as you can in 20-40 seconds in a safe manner. Always read all the notes on the *'advice on technique'* for each of the exercises in the *'exercise description'* section. This will show you how to exercise with good form, how to get results quicker and how to prevent injuries. If you feel pains in the chest or in any muscles that you are exercising; stop and seek advice.

You may feel fatigued when exercising with weights to be begin with. This will get easier throughout the program but if you start to feel immense pain, then stop! The no pain and no gain scenario is totally wrong. You will need to push yourself but in a controlled and stress free manner!

A key point to note is that the barbell exercises can be performed at a gym or you if have purchased a barbell.

However, if you don't own a barbell you can use a broom handle and perform the exercise as a bodyweight exercise. You can use all these 10 work outs at home and/or in the gym!

REST DAYS

You need your rest days for your muscles to recover properly and for you to get mentally prepared for the next work out session. As you progress through the work out plans, your body will adapt to the exercise intensity but the work outs do get gradually harder and are repeated more **(SEE PURPLE TABLE)**. You need to rest and have at least 6-8 hours of sleep, as this aids muscle growth and recover. Plus, it also enhances fat burning potential. **Good luck and Enjoy**

THE WORK OUTS

THE WARM UP

The Benefits of Doing a Warm Up

In simple terms a warm up gets you mentally and physically prepared for the work outs. It warms up the cardio vascular system properly and ensures the muscles get all of the oxygen rich blood that they require. A proper warm up can prevent injuries by preparing the muscles for the demand of the work outs. Please use this warm up before you start any of the 10 work outs.

A Simple Glossary of the Muscles Used in the Work Outs

- Core = hips, lower back and lower stomach
- Glutes = butt muscles
- Pecs = chest
- Quad = thigh muscles
- Hamstrings = upper back of leg muscles
- Tricep = back of arm muscle opposite biceps

An Outline to the Warm-Up for the Training Plans

EXERCISE	DURATION
High Knees	2 x 30 seconds
Glute Kicks	2 x 30 seconds
Lunges	2 x 30 seconds
Hip Side Kicks	2 x 30 seconds
Arm Circles	2 x 30 seconds
Leg Swings	2 x 30 seconds

THE COOL DOWN

The cool down should be performed at the end of every work out and it should be undertaken to allow your heart rate to return back to its resting levels. This routine should be completed on the recovery days if you *don't* own a foam roller.

Static Stretching

Static stretching is a very safe and effective form of stretching. There is a limited risk of injury when performed correctly and it is very beneficial for flexibility. The stretching routine should last between 5-10 minutes and should include all of the major muscle groups. Static stretching is performed by placing the body in a position whereby the muscle and tendons can be stretched under tension. Both the opposing muscle groups and the muscles to be stretched are relaxed; the body then moves to increase the tension of the muscles.

At this point the muscles are held and lengthened. The stretch should be held for about 30 seconds for maximum benefit;

remember to stretch gently/slowly, and stretch only to the point of tension. The benefits include increased flexibility and range of movement at the joints; this improvement has been associated with a reduction in injuries, especially at the hip and shoulder joints.

EXERCISE	DURATION
Hamstring Stretch	Hold for 10 seconds x 3 sets on each leg
Quad Stretch	Hold for 10 seconds x 3 sets on each leg
Tricep Stretch	Hold for 10 seconds x 3 sets on each arm
Gastrocnemius Stretch	Hold for 10 seconds x 3 sets on each leg
Kneeling Hip Flexor Stretch	Hold for 10 seconds x 3 sets on each leg
Standing Adductor Stretch	Hold for 10 seconds x 3 sets on each leg

A Roller Routine (Sundays)

A foam roller is an excellent exercise device that should be used on your recovery days. Each Sunday within the 8 week training plan has been set aside for you to follow this foam roller recovery routine. A foam roller is a foam of self-muscle tension release and it is used by many therapists to help to improvement movement, reduces muscle over activity, improves tissue and fascia extensibility and helps you to recovery properly.

There is evidence to suggest that this form of self-massage helps recovery from injuries, and it helps you to perform for longer when exercising. Foam rolling helps to improve blood flow to the muscles; this improves oxygen delivery and waste removal which is important for muscle growth, recovery and repair.

Please note that if you don't have a foam roller in your arsenal, then you can follow the cool down static stretch routine.

EXERCISE	DURATION
Rest Position	3-5 minute
Upper Back	2 minutes
Neck	1 minute
Latts	2 x 1 minute
Pecs	2 x 1 minute
Glutes/Hip Rotators	2 x 1 minute
Hamstrings	2 x 1 minute
Calves	2 x 1 minute
Hip Flexors	2 x 1 minute
Quads	2 x 1 minute
Adductors	2 x 1 minute
Shins	2 x 1 minute
Feet	2 x 1 minute

THE WORK OUTS

Some advice in terms of fitness levels:

Beginner - perform each exercise for 20 seconds with a 30 second rest in between

Intermediate - perform each exercise for 30 seconds with a 20 second rest in between

Advanced - perform each exercise for 40 seconds with a 10 second rest in between

When you advance through the 8 weeks you may want to increase the time that you are exercising and reduce the rest intervals.

These are natural fitness progressions and feel free to adjust the exercise/rest times. Try to do this by 5 seconds each because you will be surprised how much this can impact the intensity of the work outs.

You can use a Tabata timer from http://fitlb.com/tabata-timer[47], as this is free and it is excellent for adding in the timing splits of the exercises and the number of rounds (a round is 8 exercises).

In terms of the rest intervals you can either rest or jog in place - the option is yours!

Please use the purple table below to determine the number of times that you repeat the work outs. If you are finding the number of repeats too easy then work harder in the allocated time slots, as HIIT is all about working at 100% intensity.

Remember to record the number of exercises that you have performed in the work outs and use that as a target to beat in your next work out!

Week Number			
	Beginner	Intermediate	Advanced
1-4	2	3	4
5-8	3	4	5

Work Out A			
Exercise	Time	Rest	Record
Push Ups	40-20 secs	10-30 secs	
Burpees	40-20 secs	10-30 secs	
Regular Squats	40-20 secs	10-30 secs	
Forward Lunges	40-20 secs	10-30 secs	
Jacks	40-20 secs	10-30 secs	
Swiss Ball Shoulder Presses	40-20 secs	10-30 secs	
Swiss Ball Leg Raises	40-20 secs	10-30 secs	
Mountain Climbers	40-20 secs	10-30 secs	

HIIT

Work Out B			
Exercise	Time	Rest	Record
In and Out Jump Squats	40-20 secs	10-30 secs	
Mountain Climbers	40-20 secs	10-30 secs	
Opposite Arm and Leg Raises	40-20 secs	10-30 secs	
Swiss Ball Shoulders Presses	40-20 secs	10-30 secs	
Planks	40-20 secs	10-30 secs	
Spidermans	40-20 secs	10-30 secs	
Swiss Ball Dumbbell Chest Presses	40-20 secs	10-30 secs	
Lunges with Back Rows	40-20 secs	10-30 secs	

Work Out C			
Exercise	Time	Rest	Record
Bear Crawls	40-20 secs	10-30 secs	
Push Ups	40-20 secs	10-30 secs	
Squat Jumps	40-20 secs	10-30 secs	
Side Leaps	40-20 secs	10-30 secs	
Swiss Ball Jack Knifes	40-20 secs	10-30 secs	
Swiss Ball Leg Raises	40-20 secs	10-30 secs	
Upright Rows	40-20 secs	10-30 secs	
Clock Lunges	40-20 secs	10-30 secs	

HIIT

Work Out D			
Exercise	Time	Rest	Record
Ice Skaters	40-20 secs	10-30 secs	
Dumbbell Overhead Lifts	40-20 secs	10-30 secs	
Swiss Ball Dumbbell Chest Press	40-20 secs	10-30 secs	
Step Masters	40-20 secs	10-30 secs	
Swiss Ball Dumbbell Shoulder Press	40-20 secs	10-30 secs	
Burpees	40-20 secs	10-30 secs	
Forward Lunges	40-20 secs	10-30 secs	
Squat Jumps	40-20 secs	10-30 secs	

Work Out E			
Exercise	Time	Rest	Record
Log Jumps	40-20 secs	10-30 secs	
Clock Lunges	40-20 secs	10-30 secs	
Sumo Squats	40-20 secs	10-30 secs	
Opposite arm and leg raises	40-20 secs	10-30 secs	
Plank	40-20 secs	10-30 secs	
Wide Arm Push Ups	40-20 secs	10-30 secs	
Swiss Ball Jack Knifes	40-20 secs	10-30 secs	
Squat Jumps	40-20 secs	10-30 secs	

Work Out F			
Exercise	Time	Rest	Record
Burpees	40-20 secs	10-30 secs	
Goblet Squats	40-20 secs	10-30 secs	
Clock Lunges	40-20 secs	10-30 secs	
Dumbbell Overhead Lifts	40-20 secs	10-30 secs	
Hip Extensions with Reverse Fly	40-20 secs	10-30 secs	
Wide Arm Push Ups	40-20 secs	10-30 secs	
Upright Dumbbell Rows	40-20 secs	10-30 secs	
Step Masters	40-20 secs	10-30 secs	

Work Out G			
Exercise	Time	Rest	Record
Jacks	40-20 secs	10-30 secs	
Regular Squats	40-20 secs	10-30 secs	
Squat Jumps	40-20 secs	10-30 secs	
Dumbbell Overhead Lifts	40-20 secs	10-30 secs	
Lunges with Back Rows	40-20 secs	10-30 secs	
Mountain Climbers	40-20 secs	10-30 secs	
Swiss Ball Jack Knifes	40-20 secs	10-30 secs	
Swiss Ball Leg Raises	40-20 secs	10-30 secs	

HIIT

Work Out H			
Exercise	Time	Rest	Record
Tuck Jumps	40-20 secs	10-30 secs	
Goblet Squats	40-20 secs	10-30 secs	
Elevated Feet Push Ups	40-20 secs	10-30 secs	
Dumbbell Overhead Lifts	40-20 secs	10-30 secs	
Bear Crawls	40-20 secs	10-30 secs	
Swiss Ball Dumbbell Chest Presses	40-20 secs	10-30 secs	
Swiss Ball Dumbbell Shoulder Presses	40-20 secs	10-30 secs	
Jacks	40-20 secs	10-30 secs	

Work Out I			
Exercise	Time	Rest	Record
Wide Arm Push Ups	40-20 secs	10-30 secs	
Goblet Squats	40-20 secs	10-30 secs	
Bear Crawls	40-20 secs	10-30 secs	
Dumbbell Overhead Lifts	40-20 secs	10-30 secs	
In and Out Squat Jumps	40-20 secs	10-30 secs	
Elevated Feet Push Ups	40-20 secs	10-30 secs	
Lunge Jumps	40-20 secs	10-30 secs	
Plank	40-20 secs	10-30 secs	

HIIT

Work Out J			
Exercise	Time	Rest	Record
Bear Crawls	40-20 secs	10-30 secs	
Sumo Squats	40-20 secs	10-30 secs	
Spidermans	40-20 secs	10-30 secs	
Dumbbell Overhead Lifts	40-20 secs	10-30 secs	
Lunge Jumps	40-20 secs	10-30 secs	
Bulgarian Split Squats	40-20 secs	10-30 secs	
Swiss Ball Dumbbell Chest Presses	40-20 secs	10-30 secs	
Swiss Ball Dumbbell Shoulder Presses	40-20 secs	10-30 secs	

THE EXERCISE DESCRIPTIONS

This section will show and describe the exercises that make up the workout routines throughout this Chapter. All of the exercises are described in terms of how to perform them in a safe and effective manner. Don't rush this process and never neglect proper form for each of the exercises. Remember that practice really does make perfect!

WARM UP EXERCISES

ARM CIRCLES

Advice on Technique

- Standing tall with legs hip width apart and soft knees and arms down by your side

- Keep the back of your neck long, start to raise your arms out in front of you to shoulder height, continue to stretch your arms up towards the ceiling and gently backwards finishing off with your hands back down by your side

- Slowly continue with this motion, inhaling as you stretch your arms up, exhaling on return down

- Repeat in the opposite direction

- Remain tall and upright with engaged your core muscles to help support the lower back

GLUTE KICKS

Advice on Technique

- Start by standing on one leg with the other leg bent back at the knee

- Jump up switching position by bringing the planted leg up to kick the glutes and landing on the other leg

- Repeat this action

- Keep the back straight and knees soft when landing

HIGH KNEES

Advice on Technique

- Stand tall

- Lift your left arm and right leg as if you are about to run on the spot
- Keep alternating this movement raising the knees high towards the chest
- Maintain a tight core throughout the exercise by pulling your belly bottom towards the spine

HIP SIDE KICKS

Advice on Technique

- Begin by standing tall legs hip width apart
- Rest your hands on your hips for support
- Begin to extend your leg out slowly to the side raising up to hip level if capable
- Hold and gently return your leg to the start position
- Repeat five times then move on to the opposite leg
- With the stationary leg make sure that remains tall and straight, be aware not to kick out from the stationary hip
- Try not to overstrain and keep your body balanced
- You can use a wall support if needed

LEG SWINGS

Advice on Technique

- Stand sideways and hold onto a wall or a partner with right hand
- Place weight on left leg
- Swing right leg forwards and backwards from hip
- Keep your back and torsi straight
- Repeat 20 times and swap legs

LUNGES

Advice on Technique

- Begin standing tall with legs hip width apart

- Step forward with your right leg and bring the left foot on to tip toes behind you

- Start to lower your left knee to the floor making sure your right knee does not go over your right foot

- Aim for a 45 degree angle with your right leg

- Hold this position for five seconds then return your legs back to the neutral position

COOL DOWN

HAMSTRING STRETCH

Advice on Technique

- Begin by lying flat on your back on your carpet
- Slide your right heel on the floor towards your thigh, bending your leg at the knee (this helps to support)
- As you begin to raise the left leg start to lift from the shoulders and hold the back of your hamstring with your hands
- If this is too challenging have a long towel to hand and loop the towel around the back of your calve on the raised leg to help pull the leg towards your chest
- Once you have your desired hold gently pull on the towel or the back of your leg to stretch out the hamstring
- Hold this stretch for ten seconds then slowly lower your leg down to the neutral position
- Repeat on the other leg

GASTROCNEMIUS STRETCH

Advice on Technique

- Stand facing a wall
- Extend one leg back, with foot pointed straight ahead. Don't allow the rear foot to flatten.
- Bend arms and lean forward towards the wall. Keep the glute muscles and quads tight, with the heel on the ground.

- Hold for 30 seconds

KNEELING HIP FLEXOR STRETCH

Advice on Technique

- Kneel with front and back legs bent at a ninety degree angle
- Internally rotate back hip to target the inner thigh or a neutral position to target the quads
- Draw stomach inwards
- Squeeze the glute muscles of the side being stretched while rotating pelvis
- Hold for 30 seconds

QUAD STRETCH

Advice on Technique

- You may want to support yourself by placing your hand on to a wall or a chair if you feel you can't do this free standing
- Standing tall feet facing forward, legs hip width apart with soft knees
- Stretch out your right arm to the side to help balance
- Gently bend your knee bringing your heel towards your glutes
- Reach round with your left hand and hold the foot in position
- You should feel a stretch going down the front of your quad
- Keep both knees in line with one another

- Your pelvis should be slightly tilted forward which helps support the lower back

- Remain tall in your upper body

- Hold this stretch for ten seconds

- Slowly release your supporting hand from the foot and lower your foot back down to the neutral position

- Repeat on the other leg

STANDING ADDUCTOR STRETCH

Advice on Technique

- Stand in straddle position with feet shoulder width apart

- Extend one leg back until the toes of the back leg is in line with the heel of the other foot

- Both feet pointing straight ahead

- Pull stomach in and rotate pelvis

- Slowly move into a sideways lunge, until stretch in the straight leg groin is felt

- Hold for 30 seconds

TRICEP STRETCH

Advice on Technique

- This can be performed by either standing or sitting on a chair. Don't sit on the floor when performing this exercise

- Choose your desired position

- If standing have your feet facing forwards, legs hip width apart with soft knees

- If sitting, feet flat on the floor facing forwards, legs slightly apart

- Have a tall upright torso in either positions

- Start to raise your left elbow up towards the ceiling so your upper arm is parallel to the side of your temple

- Drop your arm down towards your shoulder blades

- With your right arm lift this over your head so your hand can reach the upright left elbow

- Hold the elbow and feel the stretch in the tricep

- Hold for ten seconds

- Then slowly release and return to neutral

- If this stretch is too advanced you can bring your arm across the front of your chest, making sure the shoulder does not hunch up

- With your other arm hug the stretched arm into your body to feel the stretch

- Hold for ten seconds the return to neutral

THE FOAM ROLLER EXERCISES

ADDUCTORS

Advice on Technique

- Position yourself face down on your elbows with one leg outstretched while the other leg is bent from the knee parallel with the hip joint
- Place the roller under the adductor
- Roll back and forth starting from above the knee all the way up the adductor to the groin area
- Repeat on the other adductor

CALVES

Advice on Technique

- Position the roller at the top of your calves avoiding the back of the knees
- Keep your torso upright and tall with arms placed behind you avoiding locking elbows
- Roll back and forth in small sections working your way down to the bottom of the calves
- Stretch your foot to the left and right as you roll to work either sides of the calves
- Position one ankle over the other for a more intense exercise
- Repeat on the other calf

FEET

Advice on Technique

- Position yourself by a wall standing tall
- Place one foot on the end of the roller as you support yourself by the wall with your hand
- Begin to roll your foot from heel to toe
- Gently lean your ankle to either side to massage the arch and outer-side of the foot
- Repeat on the other foot

GLUTES/HIP ROTATORS

Advice on Technique

- Position yourself sat on the roller with feet flat to the floor, knees bent and your arms outstretched behind you for balance
- Roll forward and back on the roller
- Distribute your weight from either side to target each glute
- Place right ankle above your left knee which will stretch out the right glute, roll back and forth to massage the hip rotator
- Repeat on the opposite side

HAMSTRINGS

Advice on Technique

- Position the roller at the top of the hamstrings where they meet the glutes
- Have your legs outstretched and arms placed behind you avoiding locking elbows

- Roll back and forth in small sections all the way down your hamstrings avoiding the backs of the knees

- Point your toes to the left and right as you roll to work either sides of the hamstrings

HIP FLEXORS

Advice on Technique

- Position yourself on your stomach with arms outstretched with the end of the roller under the hip flexor

- Roll back and forth onto the top of your quad and stopping just before your stomach

- Repeat on the other hip flexor

LATTS

Advice on Technique

- Position yourself on your side with the foam roller under your arm pit with the arm outstretched keeping your hand outstretched on its side

- Keep your upper leg bent at the knee with the foot flat positioned behind your lower leg for balance

- Starting from your armpit make small rolling motions gradually working down to just above the waist line

- Repeat on the other latt

NECK

Advice on Technique

- Place the roller at the base of your head

- Lay with back flat into the floor, feet flat with relaxed legs and knees bent

- Gently and slowly turn your head to either side (repeat ten times) avoiding any big movements

PECS

Advice on Technique

- Lie on your stomach with the roller placed under your pec along the side of your torso
- Roll across the roller from side to side up to ten times from your arm to your pec

QUADS

Advice on Technique

- Position yourself on your elbows face down with legs outstretched
- Place the roller under your quads (keep your core engaged to support the lower back)
- Roll back and forth on the quads
- Point the feet to the left and right to work either side of the quads
- Position one leg across the other as you roll back and forth for a more intense exercise
- Repeat on the opposite quad

REST POSITION

Advice on Technique

- Lay flat on the floor with the roller under your head supporting your spine and lower back
- Arms out to the side and place your feet flat on floor with legs

- relaxed and slightly bent at the knees
- Hold this position 3-5 minutes with deep breathing

SHINS

Advice on Technique

- Position yourself on your elbows facedown with the roller under your shins
- Using your weight on your elbows roll back and forth massaging all the area of the shins
- To work the outer part of the shins cross one leg over the other and roll on the outer side of the shin from below the knee to above the ankle
- Repeat on the other shin

UPPER BACK

Advice on Technique

- Position the foam roller under your shoulder blades , arms bent at your elbows with hands by your ears
- Engage your glutes and core
- Keeping the moves short, roll up and down the roller with your upper back
- Move your weight slightly to opposite sides to target muscles on either side of the upper back
- Do not roll below your mid-back area

EXERCISES IN WORK OUTS

BEAR CRAWLS

Advice on Technique

- Begin on your hands and knees
- Then rise up onto your toes and in a controlled manner reach forward with your left arm and left knee.
- This in turn is followed by the right side of your body and then start the crawl
- Your bodyweight is now on your hands and toes and keeping a smooth rhythm is important to maintain balance and speed of motion during exercise

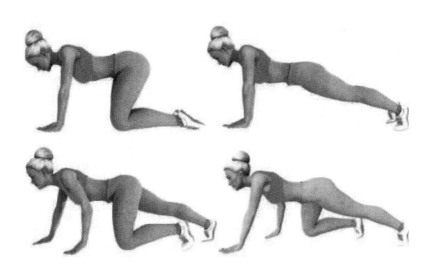

BULGARIAN SPLIT SQUATS

Advice on Technique

- Place one leg onto box or chair, with the opposite leg in contact with the floor

- Balance over opposite leg, with barbell or broom handle supported solidly on back of shoulders/bottom of neck

- Squat downwards on your weight bearing leg until your upper quad is parallel to ground

- Keep your core tight and engaged throughout whole motion of squat

- Drive bodyweight up through heels and repeat with opposite leg after 1 rep

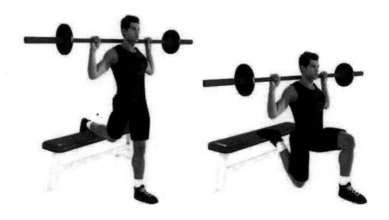

BURPEES

Advice on Technique

- Start off in the squat position with your hands placed on the floor
- Kick both feet back
- Go down into a full body push up
- Jump both feet back to return to the squat position
- Stand up and end with a jump
- Repeat
- Maintain smooth controlled motions throughout this exercise
- Keep your core tight with a straight back at all times

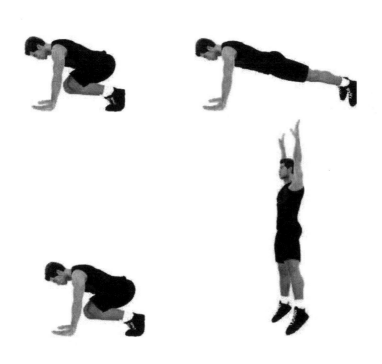

CLOCK LUNGES

Advice on Technique

- Perform a traditional forward lunge

- Then take a large step to the left and perform a lunge again

- Complete the exercise with a backwards lunge and return to the standing position and then repeat.

- Switch legs and repeat.

- Ensure your neck lines up with your spine.

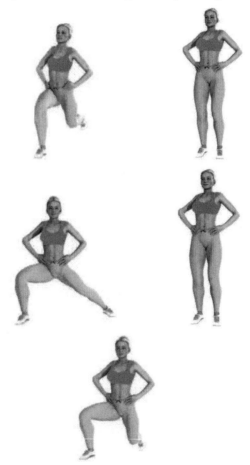

DUMBBELL OVERHEAD LIFTS

Advice on Technique

- Stand with your feet shoulder-width apart and hold dumbbell out in front with both hands
- Squat down and touch the floor with the dumbbell
- Keep your back straight and core engaged
- Return to start position and push dumbbell above your head and straighten arms
- Reset the position and repeat movement pattern

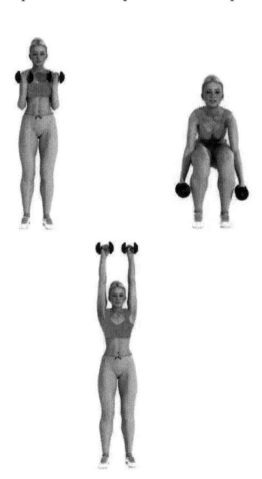

ELEVATED FEET PUSH UPS

Advice on Technique

- Place your hands shoulder-width apart on the ground

- The back of your wrists should be facing your toes and feet

- Your feet should be elevated on a platform, ball or box. The higher the box/platform/ball the more you will work your shoulders, chest, core and stabilisers

- Try to dig your toes into the box/ball/platform as this will help with balance

- Lower your chest down as close to the ground as possible

- Push back up

- Maintain a tight core at all times

- Do not let your lower back dip

- Exhale on exertion

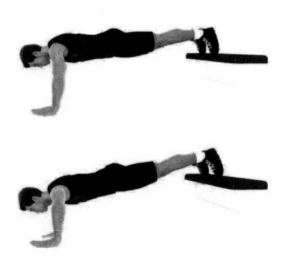

FORWARD LUNGES

Advice on Technique

- Begin standing tall with legs hip-width apart

- Step forward with your right leg and bring the left foot on to tiptoes behind you

- Start to lower your left knee to the floor making sure your right knee does not go over your right foot

- Aim for a 45 degree angle with your right leg

- Change this position by then returning your legs back to the neutral position

- Repeat quickly with alternative leg for the length of the Tabata

- Keep your back tall and straight when lowering down

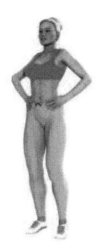 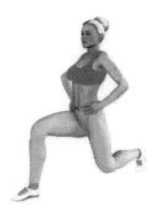

GOBLET SQUATS

Advice on Technique

- Stand up with dumbbell in front of you at chest height
- Feet just outside shoulder width apart and feet facing forwards
- Keep a tight core, flat lower torso and squat downwards
- Push your hips back up, until you are just below parallel with your knee bend
- Drive bodyweight back up through heels and engage core at all times

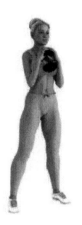 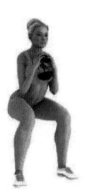

HIP EXTENSION WITH REVERSE FLY

Advice on Technique

- Use a weighted dumbbell in each hand and stand talk
- Then extend your right leg and keep it straight, your toes should always be in contact with the floor
- Lift the extended leg keeping it at hip height and move your chest towards the ground
- At the same time move your arms out straight and squeeze your shoulder blades together
- Relax your head and neck, always keeping them in line

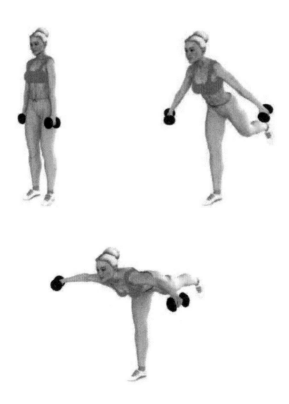

ICE SKATERS

Advice on Technique

- Stand with feet shoulder width apart and toes pointing forwards

- Rapidly push from side to side, whilst keeping the body aligned during the hopping movement

- Repeat as quickly and land on ball of feet when hopping off either foot

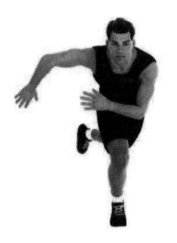 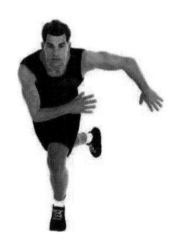

IN AND OUT JUMP SQUATS

Advice on Technique

- Start with your legs hip-width apart
- Go down in to the regular squat position
- Jump up to an outer squat
- Jump up and return to the regular squat
- Keep the movement smooth and controlled

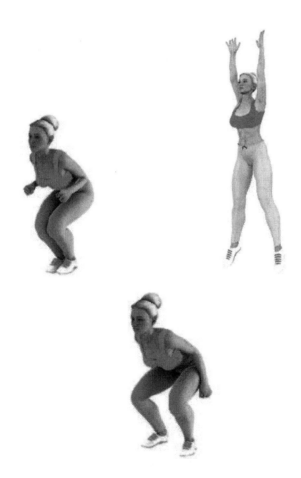

JACKS

Advice on Technique

- Start by standing tall with your arms by your side with your legs and feet together

- Power up from the legs with your arms reaching high above your head and your legs kicking out

- Bring your arms and legs back to the starting position on return

- Keep the chest open to avoid the shoulders arching

- Keep the knees soft on landing

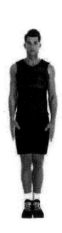
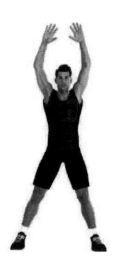

LOG JUMPS

Advice on Technique

- Start of by sprinting on the spot
- Propel your right leg up and jump over to the right side landing on your right foot
- With your left leg up propel across landing on your left foot
- Repeat
- Keep the core muscles tight and your back straight
- Put your arms out to the side to balance if needed

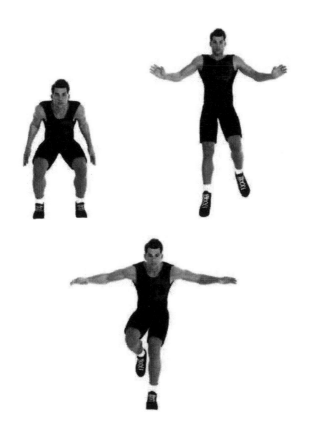

LUNGE JUMPS

Advice on Technique

- Stand with feet together and lunge in a forward motion with the right foot
- Then jump vertically by thrusting your arms upwards and by keeping your elbows bent
- When in flight switch legs and land on the ground with the opposite leg in the lunge position.
- Repeat

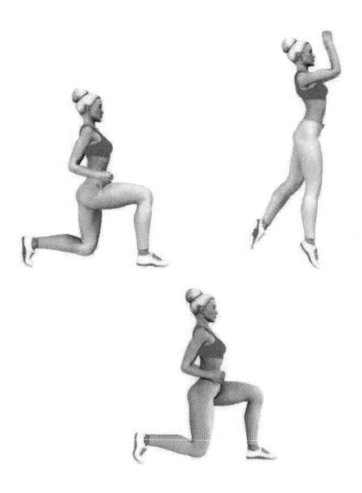

LUNGES WITH BACK ROW

Advice on Technique

- The same principle as using the forward lunge technique
- However, during the lunge downwards have the dumbbells parallel with the floor and arms straight
- On the upwards part of the lunge perform an upwards row with the dumbbells
- Engage your core throughout movement

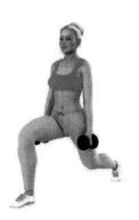 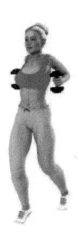

MOUNTAIN CLIMBERS

Advice on technique

- Start on all fours with your legs hip-width apart
- Arms shoulder-width apart with your hands flat on the floor
- Keep your shoulders above your wrists
- Your glutes should be slightly higher than the regular push-up position
- Bring your knee towards your chest
- Keep your knee on the inside of your arms
- Return your leg to the starting position
- Alternate legs quickly as you can
- Keep a tight core throughout the exercise
- Do not allow your back to dip

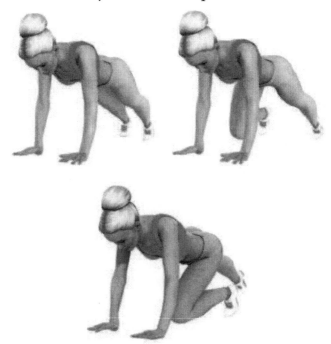

OPPOSITE ARM AND LEG RAISES

Advice on Technique

- Position yourself on all fours with elbows and wrists in line with your shoulders and knees under your hips

- Start to lift and extend your right arm out so it is parallel with your shoulder as your left leg extends and raises up to hip height

- Change this position quickly after you stretch your arm and push back into your extended heel

- Return quickly back to all fours then repeat on the other side

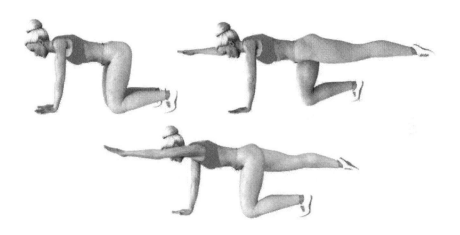

PLANKS

Advice on technique

- Lay flat on your stomach on the floor with feet together and forearms on the floor

- Lift body off the ground until it forms a straight line from head to toes, resting on your forearms and toes

- Keep back straight and chin tucked in

- Hold for 20 seconds

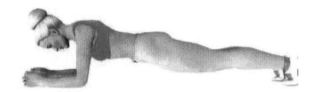

PUSH UPS

Advice on Technique

- Start in push up position
- The back of your wrists should be facing your toes and feet
- Extend your arms and stabilise wrists
- Keep your legs together and your body straight at all times
- Lower your chest down until its level with the ground or you can go as close to the ground comfortable.
- Push back up
- Repeat
- Maintain a tight core
- Do not let your lower back dip
- Exhale on upwards motion

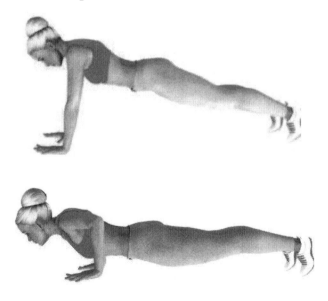

REGULAR SQUATS

Advice on Technique

- Standing tall with feet facing forward, legs hip-width apart with soft knees

- Bring both of your arms out in front of you

- Begin to lower your buttocks down as if you were going to sit back on a chair

- Keep your arms out at shoulder level, knees over ankles and thighs in line with hips

- Push back up through your feet straightening your legs back to the neutral position, bringing your arms back down to your side

- Repeat

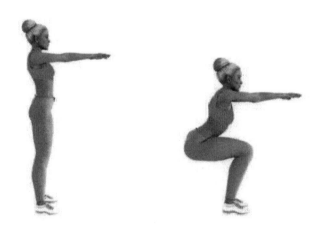

SIDE LEAPS

Advice on Technique

- Stand with feet together
- Bend your knees and hop as far as you can go with you left foot
- Land on the balls of your right foot
- Reverse action and repeat
- Drive your arms and try to get a smooth rhythm going

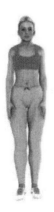 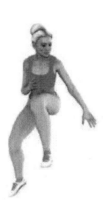

SIDE PLANKS

Advice on Technique

- Forearm on mat with shoulder and arm in one line
- Legs on top of one another
- Lift the body off the floor keeping the core tight
- Rest one hand on the hip to help with balancing the body
- Swap side once you have completed half of the allocated time

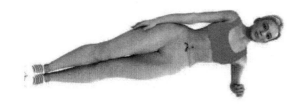

SPIDERMANS

Advice on Technique

- Start in the push up position with your body straight

- Bring your right knee up and out towards your right elbow as your left hand extends forward

- Staying low to the ground alternate your bent knee and hand as you crawl forward

- Keep your back straight throughout the exercise with a tight core

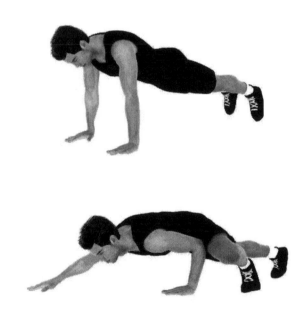

SQUAT JUMPS

Advice on technique

- Stand with your legs shoulder-width apart, hands placed at temples with elbows out to the side with your weight in the heels

- Push out your bottom as you lower your hips to 90 degrees from the floor

- Keep your knees above the ankles

- Power up through your legs and jump landing on your heels

- Keep your back straight and your core tight

- Exhale on the jump up, inhaling on the landing

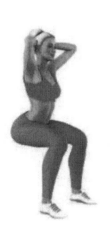 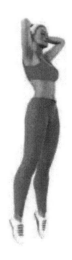

STEP MASTERS

Advice on Technique

- Begin in standing position with right foot on the bench/wall/step

- Hands together and elbows tucked in

- Drive off left foot and drive elbows through upwards, until feet are on the bench

- Maintain a solid core position

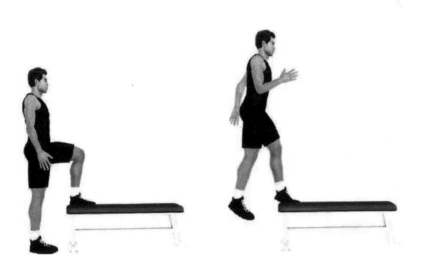

SUMO SQUATS

Advice on Technique

- Hold a dumbbells, out in front of you and in between your legs
- Have a wide stance with feet wider than shoulder width
- Feet should be facing slight outwards, and this aids balance
- Keep torso upright, back straight and move hips/dumbbell towards ground and below knee level
- Drive bodyweight back up through heels and engage core at all times

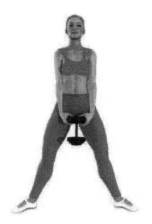 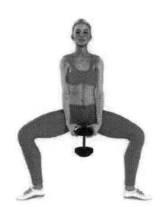

SWISS-BALL DUMBBELL CHEST PRESSES

Advice on Technique

- Have hold of light pair of dumbbells

- Position yourself on the Swiss ball with your upper and middle part of your back pressed firmly on to the ball

- Your knees should be bent with your hips raised so your body is aligned straight

- Place your arms up towards the ceiling keeping in line with your shoulders taking care not to allow them to drop backwards

- Have your palms facing forwards yet slightly turned inwards

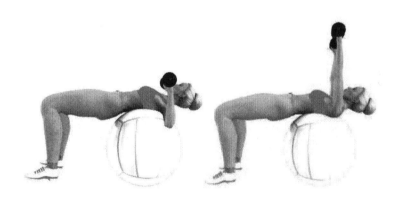

SWISS BALL DUMBBELL SHOULDER PRESSES

Advice on Technique

- Hold some light weight dumbbells
- Position your weights in your hands with the weights parallel to your shoulders and elbows pointing downwards
- Push the weights up so your arms are extended up above the shoulders
- Return your weights back down to shoulder height with the elbows down by your side

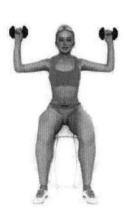 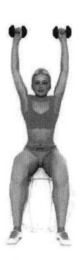

SWISS BALL JACK KNIFES

Advice on Technique

- Start in the press up position with the Swiss ball

- The ball should be in contact with the ankles and the arms holding all of the body weight.

- Roll the Swiss ball towards your hips by bending your knees, have a short pause and then return to starting position

- Exhale when rolling the Swiss ball towards the hips, and inhale in when rolling the ball back to starting position

- Through the exercise contract your core upwards your back

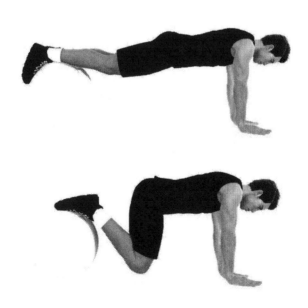

SWISS BALL LEG RAISES

Advice on Technique

- Lay on your back with the Swiss ball between your lower legs

- Hands slightly out by your side to support yourself

- Keep the stomach muscles engaged to protect your lower back

- Lift your legs with the Swiss ball until your hips are about 90 degrees

- Hold this position briefly then return your legs to the starting position

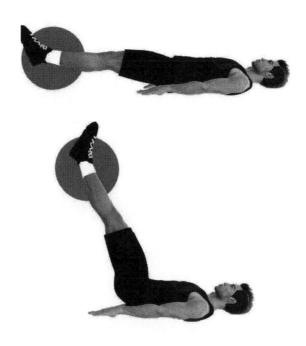

TUCK JUMPS

Advice on Technique

- Stand with feet shoulder-width apart
- Jump off the floor and when in air bring your knees to your chest
- Land softly on mid-section of foot, with feet straight and knees over the mid-section of the foot
- Like all jumps, the tuck jump should be performed with control

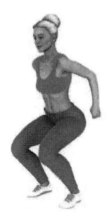 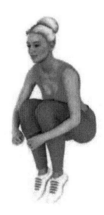

UPRIGHT DUMBBELL ROWS

Advice on Technique

- Select two dumbbells with the weight that is suitable for you

- Stand with feet at shoulder-width apart and knees slightly bent

- Lift both arms slowly sideways until your upper arms are parallel with the floor

- When your arms reach the highest point (shoulder height) hold this position and contract your upper back by tensing your shoulder blades together

- Slowly return to the neutral position

- Inhale as you lift the dumbbells

- Slowly exhale as your return to neutral

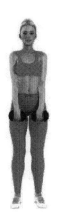 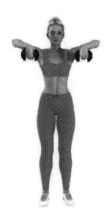

WIDE ARM PUSH UPS

Advice on Technique

- Arms wider than shoulder-width
- Keep your legs together and your body straight at all times
- Lower your chest down until it almost touches the ground
- Push your body weight back up
- Always engage your core
- Do not let your lower back dip
- Exhale on exertion

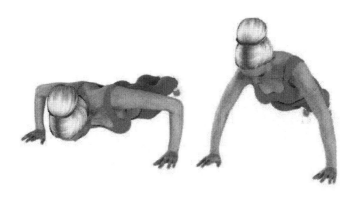

CHAPTER 5
A HEALTHY NUTRITION OUTLOOK TO USE WITH HIIT

The 'SIX-MIX' plan is a simple and easy diet to follow and it will help you to kick start your weight loss goals and aspirations. The nutrition schedule lasts for 8 weeks, and it is a positive remapping of your eating habits based around a simple concept of the number 'SIX'.

Visualise the table below and ask yourself this question 'How much weight can I lose in 8 weeks or 56 days?' The answer is on average 1-2 pounds per week or around 17 pounds in total which is a healthy range of weight loss.

This is a very healthy range of weight loss and whilst following this program, you will be losing the inches in the right places. This diet program has been designed to use in conjunction with the 10 training plans; providing a powerful combination which will definitely give your body the boost and energy that it needs to shift your unwanted weight.

HIIT

Week number	MON	TUE	WED	THU	FRI	SAT	SUN	Total Weight Loss
1	1	2	3	4	5	6	7	
2	8	9	10	11	12	13	14	
3	15	16	17	18	19	20	21	
4	22	23	24	25	26	27	28	
5	29	30	31	32	33	34	35	
6	36	37	38	39	40	41	42	
7	43	44	45	46	47	48	49	
8	50	51	52	53	54	55	56	

The Number SIX

The number 'SIX' relates to the daily amounts of your complete proteins, starches, fruits and vegetables that you need to consume. Yes, that is right - 'SIX' choices from each food group, every day for 8 weeks. That is straight forward enough and the diet model is not based around a FAD approach, but goes back to basics in terms of eating the right foods, the right portion sizes and the right timings of meals.

More importantly you will *not* feel hungry during this program because you will be eating enough of the right calories to feel satisfied and to drop the weight at the same time. Plus you will have plenty of energy to perform the 10 work outs with some real zest.

A shopping list has been created for you to choose from, and it incorporates all of the major foods that are required to help you to lose weight over the 8 week period and beyond. In addition, a food diary has been created so that you can track your food intake and reflect on any patterns of success that you throughout the course of the 8 weeks.

In addition, three meal plans have been created for you; they incorporate the foods from the shopping list along with the relevant portion sizes. The meal plans should be followed at the start of each of week and then recorded into your food diary. They should give you some ideas of how to combine the various foods, and identify the timing of the meals along with snacks. One of the main aims of all of the meal plans is to ensure that you don't feel hungry and that your metabolism remains revved up all day; ultimately to lose weight and build some lean muscle.

THE IMPORTANCE OF PORTION SIZE

Portion size is extremely important when preparing foods and 'tight plate / dish management' is crucial when dropping the weight. The following table is a guideline to portion sizes for the 'SIX-MIX' plan and you should adhere to them throughout the whole program. Once you get into the swing of portion sizing and start seeing your weight loss results; you will wonder why you have never followed this simple strategy before!

FOOD TYPES	PORTION SIZE PER MEAL
All starches	¼ of a cup
Complete Proteins	2-3 oz
Incomplete Proteins	3-4 oz
Vegetables	As much as you like
Fruit	Size of a tennis ball= 80 g Apple, pear & banana= medium fruit Plum, kiwi & Satsuma=1-2 fruits Grapes/berries= 6 – 8
Nuts	8 maximum
Seeds	1 tablespoon
Oils	1 teaspoon of oil
Calcium Rich Foods	1 x 200 ml 1 x 80 grams

THE MACROS

CARBOHYDRATES

The timing of your starches intake will be planned, so that you feel energized throughout the day, without the food cravings that come from the dreaded dips in your blood sugars. Ultimately, the right timings of the 3 types of starch intake will help you to train with real purpose whilst performing the 10 work out routines. It will also keep you on the right path for weight loss and the timings of the starch intakes are as follows:

- Resistance starches = after 3pm

- Fast starches = before a work out or in the morning

- Other starches = before 3pm

An added bonus of the 'SIX-MIX' diet is that you can eat as much vegetables as you like you from the shopping list, and you can also mix this in with some small pieces of fruits.

These food types give you all of the vital vitamins and minerals that are needed for burning fat, boosting your metabolism, reducing hunger pangs and increasing your energy levels. These micronutrients have an essential part to play in your weight loss quest and are in *abundance* on the shopping list below.

PROTEINS

Proteins are important for weight loss because they help with keeping your metabolism high, stop you from feeling hungry and aid growth / recovery after your works outs. However, to consume *all* of the essential amino acids from proteins that are required for these *key* functions, you should eat a mixture of complete and incomplete proteins.

Let's explain how this works; for example you can eat complete proteins such as oily fish from animal based proteins and / or quinoa from plant based proteins. This strategy will give you all of the essential amino acids that you require. However, another approach is to combine incomplete proteins together, and this will give you all of the essential amino acids that you need for a healthy and sustainable weight loss. These incomplete protein/s combinations are as follows:

- Legumes + nuts e.g. chick peas + tahini (sesame paste) = hummus

- Legumes + seeds e.g. lentils + chia seeds

- Legumes + grains e.g. rice and beans

Once you master how to make complete proteins, you will be well on your way to losing weight.

FATS

Not all fats are bad! Your diet plan will consist of around 15% sourced from good fats in terms of total calories consumed. The main sources of fats are from fatty fish, olive oils, nuts and seeds and not from hydrogenated and trans-fats. These oils and seeds can help to enhance your metabolism by helping to control the thyroid gland.

This can be achieved by adding one tablespoon of olive oil, rapeseed or linseed oils to your foods or to cook with them twice a day. These essential fats have the following benefits for your body:

- They are an excellent source of energy and they help to meet your daily calorie requirements

- They help with delivery and absorption of the fat soluble vitamins

- They enhance the satiety of meals and stop you from feeling hungry.

SODIUM

Salt intake will not directly relate to your weight loss but it does cause water retention. To avoid the bloated look decrease your salt intake as much as possible.

WATER

Water is vital for health maintenance, increasing your body's function and metabolism. It has an important role in weight loss and maintaining a lean body mass because it reduces your blood viscosity which helps to deliver nutrients and fat burning hormones to the working muscles. Water can help you to feel full so try to drink at least 2-3 litres per day.

MEAL TIMINGS AND SOME SUGGESTIONS

Follow these guidelines and create your meals throughout your day.

BREAKFAST

Eat within 45 minutes of getting out of bed. The body will be in a fasted state after about 8-10 hours of sleep. This fasted state can have a negative on the body which can slow down your metabolism. Your glucose levels will be decreased, along with a slower breakdown of body fat and the muscle will be in a catabolic state.

Breakfast is the most important part of the day as it gets your metabolism going, increases your body's fat burning potential and puts some fuel (glucose) back in the tank. An ideal breakfast should have a faster release carb, some protein and a small portion of good fats e.g. walnuts.

MID- MORNING SNACK

You should try to keep your blood sugars balanced and stop yourself from feeling hungry. This can be easily avoided by having a snack 2 hours after breakfast that has a fasting acting carb along with some protein.

LUNCH

Lunch is the second largest meal of the day and should be eaten 2 hours after the mid-morning snack. At this point your body should be balanced in terms of energy. The main aim of lunch is to keep your metabolism fired up and your blood sugars level. This will keep your energy levels high throughout the afternoon and should include some starches from the shopping list.

AFTERNOON SNACK

You may feel a post lunch dip in your energy and this is caused by a lag of insulin. This can be easily remedied by stabilising your blood sugars with some resistance carbs and some complete proteins.

DINNER

This is the last main meal of the day and should be consumed within 3 hours of eating your lunch. The main focus of this meal is to keep your metabolism burning with some resistance carbs, high in complete protein and a moderate fat content.

EVENING SNACK

You should aim to eat this snack 2 hours before you go to bed. It should be low in carbs, high in complete proteins and have some essential fatty acids. This will ensure that your body is still burning fat and your metabolism remains high. In addition it will increase your glycogen and proteins stores when sleeping and it will stop your muscles from going into a catabolic state.

PRE & POST WORK OUT MEALS

Adjust your breakfast, lunch or dinner to the guidelines below depending on which will precede your work outs.

PRE- WORK OUT MEALS

The main objective of the pre work-out meal is to begin training in a fed state and to ensure that all of the foods eaten have been digested properly. Therefore follow these simple guidelines with your pre-work out meals to ensure that this happens:

- Drink plenty of water to ensure that you are hydrated

- Ensure to include about 200-300 grams of fast-acting carbs for energy
- Ensure to include at least 50 g of protein to increase lean muscle mass
- Eat this meal 2-3 hours before you train

POST WORK-OUT MEALS

This meal is very important for aiding recovery along with growth and repair. A whey protein shake is an excellent supplement that can be used to facilitate these functions and it should be taken within 15 minutes of finishing your work out. It will also increase your glycogen stores. Add a banana or an orange to boost your lost electrolyte levels.

In terms of a proper meal stick to the 4:1 ratio carbs to protein and see the shopping list and the meal plans for some food/meal ideas.

FOODS TO AVOID

Avoid foods that are high in fructose, trans and hydrogenated fats. The body can't use these foods as an energy source and they are stored as unwanted body fat. These types of junk sugars and fats are associated with obesity, high blood pressure and heart disease. Always read the label and avoid the following foods:

- Milk chocolate, potato chips, pastries and pies
- Diary blends, creams, ice cream, full fat dairy and mayonnaise
- Fatty meats such as sausages, bacon and salami
- Sugary cereals
- Canned processed fats

THE SHOPPING LIST

STARCHES

STARCHES BEFORE 3 PM	RESISTANCE STARCHES AFTER 3PM	FASTER STARCHES AM OR AROUND WORK OUTS
Corn	Kidney Beans	Oatmeal
Parsnips	Black Beans	Brown Rice
Butternut Squash	Garbanzo Beans	Oats
Acorn Squash	Hummus	Wheat Pasta
Pumpkin	Beets	White Potatoes
Plantains	Amaranth	
Sweet Potato	Quinoa	
Purple Potato	Lentils	
Peas	Other Beans	
Yams		

VEGETABLES & FRUITS

VEGETABLES	FRUITS
Artichokes	**CITRUS**
Alfalfa Sprouts	
Broccoli	Grapefruit
Carrots	Oranges
Cauliflower	Limes
Celery	Lemons
Cabbage	Kumquats
Collards	Satsumas
Asparagus	Tangerines
Brussel Sprouts	Ugli Fruit
Bok Choy	**BERRIES**
Jicama	Acai Berry
Kale	Bilberry
Cucumber	Blackberry
Okra	Blueberry
Onions	Cranberry
Green Beans	Goji Berry
Mushrooms	Raspberry

VEGETABLES	FRUITS
Egg Plant	Strawberry
Spinach	**OTHER**
Peppers	Cherries
Radishes	Apples
	Kiwi
	Pineapple
	Pears
	Pomegranates
	Bananas
	Tomatoes

PROTEINS

Complete ANIMAL BASED PROTEINS	Complete PLANT BASED PROTEINS	Incomplete PROTEINS
FISH	Quinoa	**NUTS & SEEDS**
Salmon	Buck wheat	Almonds
Mackerel	Hemp seeds	Walnuts
Tuna	Chia seeds	Cashews
Rainbow Trout		Pistachios
Halibut		
Lobster		Pumpkin
Sardines		Sunflower
Herring		Flaxseeds
POULTRY		**LEGUMES**
Skinless chicken breast		Kidney Beans
Skinless turkey breast		Black Beans
		Lentils
LEAN MEATS		

Complete ANIMAL BASED PROTEINS	Complete PLANT BASED PROTEINS	Incomplete PROTEINS
Lean beef cuts		
Lean pork loins		
DAIRY		
Eggs		
Fat free Greek yoghurt		
Skimmed milk		
Low fat cottage cheese		

SAMPLE MEAL PLANS

SAMPLE MEAL PLAN 1

Breakfast	Berry Banana Oatmeal ¼ Cup of Oatmeal with 120mls of skimmed milk or soy milk Add ½ a chopped banana and 4 berries of your choice
Mid-morning	6 pistachio nuts & 1 apple
Lunch	Baked Potato with Mackerel and Rainbow Salad Small baked purple potato or sweet potato with 3oz of fresh mackerel (fish of your choice) Served on a bed of spinach, ¼ cup corn, chopped yellow and red peppers, chopped red onion, 1table spoon of dry fried pumpkin seeds 1 tea spoon of olive oil and vinaigrette dressing (mix together as a dressing)
Mid-afternoon	80 grams of low fat Greek yogurt with 1 chopped kiwi fruit mixed in.
Dinner	Pork Loin with Blood Orange, Beet and Quinoa Salad Grill 3oz of pork tender loin Severed with ¼ cup of cooked quinoa mixed and ¼ cup of beets

	Add ½ a chopped blood orange and 2 chopped kumquats into the quinoa/beets, season to taste
Mid-evening	Hummus with Dips ¼ cup hummus served with celery, carrot and cucumber sticks

SAMPLE MEAL PLAN 2

Breakfast	Oatmeal and Nutty Banana Smoothie ¼ cup oatmeal, ½ banana, 4 chopped walnuts (nut of your choice) blended with 200ml skimmed or soy meal
Mid-morning	2 plums and 6 almonds
Lunch	Curried Turkey Salad Grill a 3oz turkey and then chop up. Mix with 80 grams of low fat Greek yogurt and ½ teaspoon curry powder Then freshly squeeze a lime into the Greek yogurt Slice 8 grapes in half and chop up 6 cashew nuts, Then slice up a celery stick and one whole red onion Then serve on a bed of spinach, chopped tomato, peppers Sprinkle 1 tea spoon of sesame seeds over the top
Mid-afternoon	6 grapes 4 brazil nuts

Dinner	Fish with Lentils
	Steam 3oz of fish of your choice.
	Serve on a bed of ¼ cup cooked green lentils with sautéed mushroom, onions.
	Steam some broccoli, carrots, cauliflower, add 1 tea spoon of chia seeds over the top
Mid-evening	80 g of low fat cottage cheese mix with 4 cherries

SAMPLE MEAL PLAN 3

Breakfast	Boiled egg with Asparagus
	1 large soft boiled egg with 4 sprigs steamed asparagus
Mid-morning	½ grapefruit and 4 Brazil nuts
Lunch	Chicken with Black Bean and Brown Rice
	Grill 3oz chicken breast,
	Add ¼ cup of brown cooked rice mixed with 3oz cooked black beans, lightly sautéed mushroom and spring onions
	Mix with garlic in 1 teaspoon olive oil
Mid-afternoon	¼ cup hummus with sliced carrots and peppers, chunks of raw cauliflower
Dinner	Quinoa Stuffed Pepper with Fresh Green Salad
	1baked pepper stuffed with 3oz quinoa, sautéed garlic, mushrooms and onions mix with 1 tea spoon of olive oil.
	Served with a green leaf salad spinach, alfalfa sprouts, chopped celery 1 teas spoon of sesame seeds, and 1 tea spoon of vinaigrette dressing
Mid-evening	80g of low Greek Yogurt and 4 cherries

Steve Ryan

FOOD DIARY

Make a copy of this food diary for the 8 weeks to track your diet and eating habits throughout the training. Remember to add all of the food that you have eaten and include the portion amounts e.g. lean proteins 2-3oz. The food diary is an excellent reflective tool and will keep you on the right path throughout your weight loss journey.

	MON	TUES	WED	THU	FRI	SAT	SUN	NOTES relating to Goals
Breakfast Half hour after waking up								
Mid Morning Snack 2 hours after breakfast								
Lunch 2/3 hours after mid morning snack								
Mid Afternoon Snack 2 hours after lunch								

	MON	TUES	WED	THU	FRI	SAT	SUN	NOTES relating to Goals
Dinner 2 hours after mid afternoon snack								
Mid Evening Snack 2/3 hours after dinner								
Fluids								

AND FINALLY, SOME WEIGHT LOSS TIPS

The following section has some excellent weight loss tips to use while undertaking the 8 week program.

Carry Healthy Snacks

Always have healthy snacks on your person such as fruit and nuts. This stops you from eating junk foods and will help to maintain your blood sugars.

Shop on a Full Stomach

When you are buying the foods from the shopping list ensure that you shop on a full stomach. This will help that you stick to buying the foods on the list and you will be less likely to fill your trolley with junk foods.

Eat Slowly

You eat far less calories if you sit down properly and eat your meal slowly. When rushing your food it sends mixed signals to the brain and you will not feel full after eating your meal. This will ensure that you don't overeat and start to snack once you finish your meal.

Caffeine

Limit your intake to 2 cups of coffee per day. Coffee can help to suppress your appetite and can increase your fat burning potential. Use skimmed or soy, almond or coconut milk.

Green Tea

This is an excellent substitute for tea and coffee. It contains EGCG which is a superb fat burner because it boosts your metabolism by increasing your core body temperature.

Spice up your Meals

Add some hot peppers or some chilli powder as this contains capsaicin. These compounds increase your body temperature and metabolism which is an excellent strategy for torching fat.

Have a Good Night's Sleep

Having a good night's sleep is important for your mental and physical health. A quality sleep of around 8 hours can improve glycogen metabolism and increase your human growth hormone levels which are important fat burning hormone. Cortisol levels are also controlled with a quality sleep and this stress hormone is a major fat storing hormone.

Moderate Alcohol Intake

Be sensible when drinking alcohol because it is full of empty calories, stops the absorption of fat soluble vitamins and is a major catalyst for gaining weight. It also reduces muscular strength and tone.

ENDNOTES

[0]http://www.ncbi.nlm.nih.gov/pubmed?term=Talanian
%20JL%5BAuthor
%5D&cauthor=true&cauthor_uid=17170203

[1]http://www.ncbi.nlm.nih.gov/pubmed?term=Galloway
%20SD%5BAuthor
%5D&cauthor=true&cauthor_uid=17170203

[2]http://www.ncbi.nlm.nih.gov/pubmed?term=Heigenhauser
%20GJ%5BAuthor
%5D&cauthor=true&cauthor_uid=17170203

[3]http://www.ncbi.nlm.nih.gov/pubmed?term=Bonen%20A
%5BAuthor%5D&cauthor=true&cauthor_uid=17170203

[4]http://www.ncbi.nlm.nih.gov/pubmed?term=Spriet%20LL
%5BAuthor%5D&cauthor=true&cauthor_uid=17170203

[5]http://www.ncbi.nlm.nih.gov/pubmed/17170203/

[6]http://www.ncbi.nlm.nih.gov/pubmed?term=Talanian
%20JL%5BAuthor
%5D&cauthor=true&cauthor_uid=17170203

[7]http://www.ncbi.nlm.nih.gov/pubmed?term=Galloway
%20SD%5BAuthor
%5D&cauthor=true&cauthor_uid=17170203

[8]http://www.ncbi.nlm.nih.gov/pubmed?term=Heigenhauser
%20GJ%5BAuthor
%5D&cauthor=true&cauthor_uid=17170203

[9]http://www.ncbi.nlm.nih.gov/pubmed?term=Bonen%20A
%5BAuthor%5D&cauthor=true&cauthor_uid=17170203

[10]http://www.ncbi.nlm.nih.gov/pubmed?term=Spriet%20LL%5BAuthor%5D&cauthor=true&cauthor_uid=17170203

[11]http://www.ncbi.nlm.nih.gov/pubmed/17170203/

[12]http://www.ncbi.nlm.nih.gov/pubmed/8897392

[13]http://link.springer.com/article/10.2165/00007256-200838020-00003

[14]http://link.springer.com/journal/40279/38/2/page/1

[15]http://search.ebscohost.com/login.aspx?direct=true&profile=ehost&scope=site&authtype=crawler&jrnl=15550265&AN=43913451&h=TiEhECuGm64gWRmWrrGi8bx3cnjO0qZfjNHwVZoMpem27oUY4IVXet2oSm02lDHMnpDNvbcjj927OC4AqYMtsg%3D%3D&crl=c

[16]http://journals.lww.com/nsca-jscr/toc/2008/05000

[17]http://books.google.com/books?id=L4aZIDbmV3oC&pg=PA204

[18]http://en.wikipedia.org/wiki/International_Standard_Book_Number

[19]http://en.wikipedia.org/wiki/Special:BookSources/978-0-7817-4991-6

[20]http://www.cdc.gov/nchs/nhanes.htm

[21]http://www.ncbi.nlm.nih.gov.myaccess.library.utoronto.ca/pubmed/21868679

[22]http://www.ncbi.nlm.nih.gov/pubmed/17414804

[23]http://www.ncbi.nlm.nih.gov/pubmed?term=Wisl%C3%B8ff%20U%5BAuthor%5D&cauthor=true&cauthor_uid=17001221

[24]http://www.ncbi.nlm.nih.gov/pubmed?term=Nilsen%20TI%5BAuthor%5D&cauthor=true&cauthor_uid=17001221

[25]http://www.ncbi.nlm.nih.gov/pubmed?term=Dr%C3%B8yvold%20WB%5BAuthor%5D&cauthor=true&cauthor_uid=17001221

[26]http://www.ncbi.nlm.nih.gov/pubmed?term=M%C3%B8rkved%20S%5BAuthor%5D&cauthor=true&cauthor_uid=17001221

[27]http://www.ncbi.nlm.nih.gov/pubmed?term=Sl%C3%B8rdahl%20SA%5BAuthor%5D&cauthor=true&cauthor_uid=17001221

[28]http://www.ncbi.nlm.nih.gov/pubmed?term=Vatten%20LJ%5BAuthor%5D&cauthor=true&cauthor_uid=17001221

[29]http://www.ncbi.nlm.nih.gov/pmc/articles/PMC1724199/

[30]http://jap.physiology.org/content/97/5/1591.full

[31]http://www.tandfonline.com/action/doSearch?action=runSearch&type=advanced&searchType=journal&result=true&prevSearch=%2Bauthorsfield%3A(Laforgia%2C+J)

[32]http://www.tandfonline.com/action/doSearch?action=runSearch&type=advanced&searchType=journal&result=true&prevSearch=%2Bauthorsfield%3A(Withers%2C+R+T)

[33]http://www.tandfonline.com/action/doSearch?
action=runSearch&type=advanced&searchType=journal&res
ult=true&prevSearch=%2Bauthorsfield%3A(Gore%2C+C+J)

[34]http://books.google.com/books?
id=L4aZIDbmV3oC&pg=PA204

[35]http://en.wikipedia.org/wiki/International_Standard_Book
_Number

[36]http://en.wikipedia.org/wiki/Special:BookSources/978-0-
7817-4991-6

[37]http://en.wikipedia.org/wiki/Journal_of_Applied_Physiolo
gy

[38]http://www.ingentaconnect.com/content/nrc/apnm/2008/0
0000033/00000006/art00010

[39]http://en.wikipedia.org/wiki/Applied_Physiology,_Nutritio
n,_and_Metabolism

[40]http://www.muscleandperformancemag.com/training/201
2/7/power-hiit

[41]http://europepmc.org/abstract/MED/8744258

[42]http://jap.physiology.org/search?author1=S.+E.
+Gordon&sortspec=date&submit=Submit

[43]http://jap.physiology.org/search?author1=W.+J.
+Kraemer&sortspec=date&submit=Submit

[44]http://jap.physiology.org/search?author1=N.+H.
+Vos&sortspec=date&submit=Submit

[45]http://jap.physiology.org/search?author1=J.+M.
+Lynch&sortspec=date&submit=Submit

[46]http://jap.physiology.org/search?author1=H.+G.
+Knuttgen&sortspec=date&submit=Submit

[47]http://fitlb.com/tabata-timer

Printed in Poland
by Amazon Fulfillment
Poland Sp. z o.o., Wrocław

Dear Darragh
Happy

The Woogle Squy3x

& The Sprockerdor

The Woogle & The Sprockerdor

Squiz Gordon

First paperback edition September 2021

Book design & illustrations by Jenn Matthews.
'Texture 48' used on cover by Ellenvd is licensed under CC BY 2.0

ISBN (paperback)
ISBN (ebook)

www.JennMatthews.com

DEDICATION

This book was heavily encouraged by my wife
Sarah—AKA 'Mum'—who was desperate for me to
write some short stories about our fur-kids. I guess
it's dedicated to her, and of course, the stars of the
show, Whisper, Dana, and Cooper.

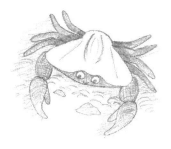

Contents

Acknowledgements

Thank you to all my amazing Beta readers: Teddy, Aoife, Bo, Paddy, & Ruby. Thank you to my proof-reader, Ann—AKA Grandma, AKA Mummy Matthews—whose exceptional grammar skills and keen eye have picked up on all my mistakes.

Thank you to Ellenvd for the 'Texture 48' background I have used on my cover. It fit so well with my illustrations.

Finally, thank you to my gorgeous fur-kids. They may occasionally cause Poo-mageddon in our kitchen, but their antics and the love they fill our house with are always worth the mopping.

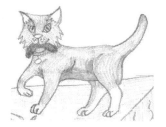

CHAPTER 1

Whisper's New Brother

hisper was a highly specialised, stripy, brown Woogle who lived with her Mama, Mum, and little sister Dana, who was a cat. She had reached the ripe old age of ten and thought that was a satisfactory age to be.

One morning, Whisper woke to find Mama and Mum in excited moods. What was happening today? Whisper couldn't remember. She knew it was something Wag—the Woogle word for 'happy'—but the 'what' was an issue. Whisper's memory had never been good; she only had three brain cells and two of them were in her tail.

Then she remembered. Today was the day her brother would be coming home to live with Whisper, Mum and Mama, who were her Hooman parents, and Dana the cat. Their family would go from four to five.

Whisper felt Wag about that. She had met her brother and he seemed very pleasant. A slow puppy who was green in colour. He appeared to eat mostly lettuce, but Whisper had loved him right away when she had met him. He'd seemed to love her back too. The perfect brother, in her eyes.

So Whisper had her morning kibble and morning Ablutions outside, then said goodbye to Mum and Mama as they left the house to travel to the Hull of Soli to collect him. Whisper settled onto the sofa and had some snore-filled Sleeps.

Several hours later, the noise of the front door opening woke Whisper from a dream about Biz Kits with a jolt. She got down from the sofa—she needed to stretch and wake up her Old Lady Legs because they had become stiff—and went to greet everyone.

Mum was carrying a very big bag. The bag smelled of kibble and puppy, but not the same puppy Whisper had met when she had visited to choose one.

Mama was carrying a dark brown puppy with huge feet and floppy ears. He didn't smell like the puppy Whisper had chosen either.

As far as Whisper could remember, her new brother was supposed to be green. He was supposed to carry his house on his back, move slowly, and eat lettuce. He was not supposed to have long ears, or ears at all actually, or brown fur, or a worm-thin tail.

Mama told Whisper her new brother was called Cooper. That was wrong too. The puppy Whisper had chosen was called Ben.

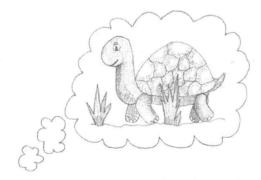

Whisper was very confused. Had Mum and Mama brought home the wrong puppy? Would they need to go back to the place the puppies came from and swap this 'Cooper' puppy for the one called Ben?

Cooper was taken outside into the garden for Wees. Mum called Whisper out to supervise. It was a lovely summer's day. Birds sang in the trees at the back and the sun was shining, making the water in the birdbath sparkle.

Whisper spent many minutes checking Cooper. She smelled his bottom, his feet, and looked several times for the house he should be carrying on his back.

Cooper walked around the garden for a while, sniffing various things, a Flou-flou here, a bit of mud there, then did a squat and some Wees.

Whisper sat thoughtfully, regarding him with a mature eye. Perhaps Ben had been chosen by another family. Perhaps Cooper had been Mum and Mama's second choice.

She couldn't ask Mum and Mama because they didn't speak Woogle. Which was a shame because Whisper could have had some very stimulating and educational conversations with her parents if they all spoke the same language.

After wagging his tail and chasing a leaf, Cooper waddled over to Whisper. "Hello."

"Hello," said Whisper. She cocked her head at him. "You're the wrong puppy."

"Am I? Ooh." Cooper plonked his bottom down and gave Whisper a worried look. "I'm so sorry."

"Hm." Whisper sat too. "Whisper can only assume that Mum and Mama chose a different puppy after Whisper chose Ben. Ben was Whisper's favourite puppy. He was green and ate lettuce. Whisper thought Ben was going to be Whisper's new brother."

"I've been informed that *I* am your brother," said Cooper. "As far as I know, Ben is a tortoise and he belongs to Daddy Ken and Daddy Gavin."

"Hmm." Whisper considered this issue. Perhaps Mum and Mama had changed their minds after all.

Then that was that. As Ben appeared to be remaining with Daddy Ken and Daddy Gavin, Cooper would have to be Whisper's new brother.

"Welcome to the place where we live," said Whisper. "Although Whisper's house is for Whisper, and therefore Cooper will have to find his own house to have Sleeps in."

"Ooh." Cooper's tongue hung out for a minute, then slurped back into his mouth. "Ya. I've got my own house. It's in the kitchen, with my Bally-ballys and my kibble and my Ducky."

"How many siblings is Whisper having?" asked Whisper, who was wondering where she was going to keep a Ducky as well as a puppy brother. Did Ducky need a pond? Whisper was not a fan of ponds.

"My Ducky is a soft toy Ducky," said Cooper. "He's very Wag and snuggly. I like snuggles."

"Whisper likes snuggles too." A toy Ducky was preferable. Whisper didn't think she could cope looking after a puppy *and* a Ducky.

Mum and Mama brought them back inside and they all went into the kitchen to check out Cooper's new area. Whisper was surprised to find a small house, far too small for Whisper, with a door on the front and a bed inside. It looked to be the correct size for Cooper, who was very small. Ducky was yellow and fluffy and looked as if it could do with some chewing and destroying.

They all went into the living room. Cooper's eyes kept closing and his little fluffy head kept nodding forward. He lay down on the carpet and put his chin on his paws. A huge sigh puffed from him. Then he yawned.

From underneath the dining table, a low growly-meow sounded. Whisper went over and stuck her nose under the table. "Hello, Dana," she said. "Have you met our new brother, Cooper?"

"What?" Dana's haughty voice made Cooper lift his head. "Brother? What?"

"This is Cooper," said Whisper, hoping Dana would be kind to him but knowing there was little chance of it. "He is a puppy but he's not Ben. Which Whisper has decided is okay."

"A new puppy? Why wasn't I informed?" Various rude words in Puzzer language fell from her mouth.

Whisper winced. "He's very small and a baby, so we have to be nice big sisters to him."

Dana made another low growl-meow. "I don't like it. It is smelly. I will smack it!"

"Well…" Whisper glanced at Cooper, who was staring at Dana and shivering a bit with fright. "It might be best not to smack him. He's staying, whether you smack him or not, and Mum and Mama might get upset if you hurt their new puppy."

"Meh." Dana's tail flopped one way, then the other, a clear indication she was not impressed. "I don't care. I'm my own Puzzer cat and no one will stop me doing my own thing."

"She's harmless really," Whisper told Cooper. "She might smack you, but her claws will be inside her paws and it won't hurt."

Cooper's eyes became rounder despite the reassurance.

8

"I'm a trained assassin," said Dana, "and I refuse to be disrespected!"

Whisper sighed. As usual, she would be the one to keep the peace.

Dana crept out from underneath the table before shooting out of the cat-flap. Cooper looked on, his eyes still like dinner plates.

"I would like to be her Fwen, if that's okay," he said. Fwen was the Woogle word for 'friend'. "I want to be everybody's Fwen because I'm a good boy."

"Whisper's sure you'll make lots of other Fwens," said Whisper. "When we go for walkies, there'll be other doggies to play with. S'lovely."

"It's lovely?" asked Cooper.

"Yeah," she replied. "S'lovely."

CHAPTER 2

That's Not What Woogles Do

After a disturbed night where Whisper had to sort out some kind of poo explosion in Cooper's house, and Mama had needed to wash all of Cooper's bedding and his Ducky because they were now brown, everyone got up to begin their first full day as a family of five.

Cooper had been bathed too. He now smelled like Shampoop and not of puppy poo, which meant that Mama and Mum were more willing to give him cuddles.

Now that Whisper had come to terms with the fact that Cooper was her brother, she was very interested in the things he did. Some of the things he did were the same as the things Whisper did. He did a little bow when he wanted to play, he chased a Bally-bally across the floor, and he liked to eat Biz Kits.

But other things he did were completely unWoogle. He slept a lot, bounded around a lot, which was frankly annoying to Whisper, and ate four times a day instead of the usual two times, at breakfast and Dindins.

Never mind; Whisper still loved him. Cooper's Ducky had come out of the tumble-dryer squeaky-clean after the poo explosion incident (which appeared to have happened because Cooper wasn't used to being left alone at night in his new house) and Whisper was excited to play tug with him.

However, Cooper seemed content to walk around in circles with Ducky in his mouth. This was not regular Woogle behaviour as far as Whisper was concerned.

Once Mum and Mama had made steaming cups of Morning Gubble Espresso and had taken these into the living room, Whisper decided to bring up this Im-paw-tant issue with him. "You're doing it wrong," said Whisper. "Toys are there to be ripped apart. Ducky needs a Fluff-ectomy. It's Woogle law."

"I don't know what a Fluff-ectomy is," said Cooper once he'd put Ducky down. "And I don't want to be a criminal."

Whisper sat neatly and pointed her nose at the ceiling in a knowledgeable way. "It's where you do a very complicated, medical procedure and remove the fluff from inside a toy."

"Ooh." Cooper looked down at Ducky with big, unsure eyes. "Ya."

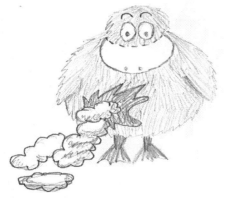

As it turned out, Cooper was quite skilled at Ducky surgery. He ripped the side of Ducky's belly open then began to pull out the cloud-like fluff. The living room carpet looked as if it had been snowed on.

But instead of cheering, or helping Cooper fulfil his Woogle duty, Mum and Mama made shouting noises and took Ducky away from Cooper.

Cooper lay down, his big paws over his nose. "I don't think I'm good at Fluff-ectomies," he said, downheartedly. "I'm not a good boy."

After licking his long floppy ear, Whisper sighed. "Don't worry, Coop. Sometimes Hoomans do things that are very confusing."

Now she considered it, it wasn't only the things Cooper *did* that were different. Cooper didn't *look* a lot like Whisper either, with his floppy ears and long fur, and his lack of stripes. He had bigger feet too, even though he was smaller than Whisper.

"Whisper has a question," said Whisper, sitting in front of Cooper.

"Ya?" Cooper wagged his tail.

"Whisper would like to know what breed Cooper is. Because Whisper is a Woogle but Cooper does things that Woogles very much do not do."

"Ooh." Cooper seemed to consider this. "I think I might be a Sprockerdor."

"What's that?" asked Whisper.

"My Mummy-dog is part Labrador and part Springer Spaniel," said Cooper, "and my Daddy-dog is a Cocker Spaniel."

"Goodness Whisper," said Whisper, "that's almost as many breeds as Whisper. Whisper has four breeds in Whisper but Whisper can never remember what they are because Whisper only has three brain cells and two are in Whisper's tail. But Whisper knows Whisper's breed is a Woogle."

"Ooh."

"What's your Daddy-dog like?"

Cooper sighed and put his head on his paws. "I never met my Daddy-dog. He only visited my Mummy-dog to get married and then he left the family to seek his fortune."

"Oh, Whisper's goodness!" Whisper jumped to her feet and lay down next to Cooper. "Whisper never met Whisper's Daddy-dog either!"

15

"So we have something in common, even if I am a Sprockerdor, and you're a Woogle?"

"Yeah." Whisper snuggled her nose against his head. "And that's S'lovely."

"It's lovely," replied Cooper as he closed his eyes and leant against Whisper's side.

CHAPTER 3

Fleshy Prince Boots

Over the next few months, Cooper grew into an adult Sprockerdor. He stopped having Wees inside, learnt various tricks and commands from Mum and Mama, and started eating two meals a day instead of four.

He was nearly the same size as Whisper, which he was pleased about. He'd felt terribly silly having Plays with Whisper because she'd had to lie on the floor so he could reach. It had been embarrassing having Wees in the kitchen when he was supposed to be having Wees in the garden.

And he never wanted to mention poo explosions again.

He was even big enough to go Swimmy-swims in the lake close to their home. He found he loved water, splashing about and generally making a commotion. He tried endlessly to coax Whisper into the lake, but she told him that a Woogle was more of a land mammal and that she was fine on the grass, thank you very much.

He got the impression he wasn't the most stylish swimmer by the way Mum and Mama laughed when he did Swimmy-swims. His paws flapped in front of him, and he held his head high out of the water. He didn't care. Swimmy-swims were too much fun.

Mum and Mama would throw sticks into the lake and he would bring them back. He discovered he was very skilled at Retrieval Services—anything Mum or Mama threw for him, he collected and brought back in record time. He could even jump into the air and catch his Bally-bally if Mum launched it high enough.

One morning during Walkies, Cooper emerged from the lake with a terrible pain in his paw. He held it up and hopped about on his three other feet until Mum came over and held out her hand.

Her voice was calming, and Cooper knew she would make him feel better. He didn't like the way his paw felt or the way it made him hop about.

Whisper came over from destroying a stick (as sticks were like toys in Woogle law; they existed to be destroyed) and cocked her head. "What's going on? Why are you walking in a strange way, Coop?"

"My paw hurts."

"Oh, Whisper's goodness! What happened?"

"I don't know. I was having Swimmy-swims and I got out of the lake and my paw hurt."

"Mum will fix it." Whisper nodded with an air of superiority and knowledge. "Mum can fix anything."

There was red stuff coming out of Cooper's paw. Mum seemed worried and snapped on their leads and took them both home. Cooper was sad as he didn't feel as if the Walkies were over, but Mum was in charge and would know what to do about his paw.

Once they'd both had a shower under the hose in the garden (Whisper being less than impressed with this state of affairs), Cooper was taken into the kitchen, still holding up his paw and hopping about on three legs.

Whisper lay down next to him and snuggled her nose against his. "Whisper's medical opinion is that you have cut your paw on something sharp."

"Ooh." Cooper looked forlornly at his paw and tried to turn it over to inspect the pad. He felt a great urge to Lup-lup his paw but stopped after Mum told him, "No."

Mum washed his paw with a liquid that smelled horrible. His paw hurt even more so Cooper made a whining noise to let Mum know. Mum ruffled his ears and used a gentle voice. That made Cooper feel better.

Once his paw was clean, Mum put soft padding against the place red stuff was coming from and wrapped a stretchy, sticky bandage around it.

The stretchy, sticky bandage was pink. "Pink is such a manly colour," thought Cooper happily.

"You won't be allowed to go Swimmy-swims with that on," said Whisper. "It will get wet, and then Mum will have to put on a new bandage."

Cooper let out a long sigh and leant into Whisper's side. "That doesn't sound very Wag." He Lup-luped the bandage because it itched.

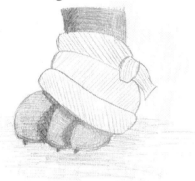

"Blimey Whisper," said Whisper. "Whisper thinks you should leave it alone. Otherwise, Mum will put the Donut of Shame on you, and you'll be bumping into things for the foreseeable future."

"Ooh," said Cooper. "Ya." He put his chin on his remaining, unbandaged paw and looked with sorrowful eyes at Mum.

Mum seemed satisfied that Cooper would be a good boy and went to tap on her iBone.

Cooper wasn't allowed to go on Walkies for a few days which made him very bored. He kept having Zoomies around the house, which Mum and Mama told him off for. He was feeling miserable.

Four days after he'd hurt his paw, a package was delivered by Nice Post Lady. Whisper always barked at her, but Nice Post Lady still smiled and said, "Hello, my friend," to Cooper.

Mum opened the package and took out four very strange items. She sat on the floor and showed them to Cooper.

Whisper came to inspect them too. "Whisper had those once," said Whisper, "they're boots like Mum and Mama wear for when you have a bad paw or foot."

"Ooh. Ya." Cooped cocked his head at them. "They are very beautiful." The boots were black and lime green. They had rubber soles and Velcro straps around the top.

"Whisper saw some exceptionally similar on the telly once. Whisper can't remember the programme, but it was something about Well Hair and a Fleshy Prince."

"I think I might have seen that when Mama was making the telly change lots," said Cooper.

Mum took Cooper's bad paw and gently slid the boot onto it over the bandage. She pulled the Velcro straps around his wrist and fastened the boot securely. Then she did the same with his non-bad paw.

Apparently just for good measure, Mum put the remaining boots on Cooper's back feet as well, so he was wearing all four of them.

"They feel awfully strange," said Cooper, lifting each paw and foot off the ground in turn and taking some tentative steps.

Whisper appeared to be holding back some kind of comment. She was looking round the kitchen at everything that wasn't Cooper and wagging her tail slowly.

Announcing her presence with her usual meow, Dana stalked into the kitchen. She stopped dead. Her eyes became round. Then she burst into Puzzer Cat laughter.

Cooper poked out his bottom lip and put all his paws and feet on the floor again. He stood tall, held his tail high, and tried to ignore the Cat-cophony coming from the other end of the kitchen.

Whisper put her face under her paws, and her whole body shook with chuckles.

"Do the boots make me look silly?" asked Cooper, disappointment swirling inside him.

"Just a tiny bit," replied Whisper, removing her paws and giving him an apologetic look.

"Oh, my goodness." Cooper lay down and sighed a big, deep sigh. "Is the Fleshy Prince not a fashion icon?"

"Whisper thinks the Fleshy Prince was probably a fashion icon thirty years ago," said Whisper. "From what Whisper has seem, he seemed a very lovely young fellow, with curly hair, and a lot of jokes." She smiled. "Mama used to laugh at the telly programme all the time."

"Ooh." Cooper considered his situation. If the Fleshy Prince was from a place called Well Hair, it probably wasn't only his boots that were fashionable; his hair must be too. And Cooper quite liked the idea of looking like a funny man from somewhere called Well Hair.

So, up Cooper clambered again and began to try out the boots properly. He still felt silly, but he pretended he was a cool, fashion icon from before he was born.

He pranced around like one of the ponies he'd seen on the beach, lifting his feet extra high. He lifted his chin and tail extra high too, to round off the look.

Dana continued to laugh, rolling onto her back and exposing her white bloomers to the world.

When Mum and Mama saw him, they clapped and laughed, which made Cooper feel better still.

"I'm the Fleshy Prince, a fashion icon," announced Cooper, his tail wagging hard enough to smack his bottom both sides, "and I have very fashionable Well Hair!"

CHAPTER 4

Magical Wags

Mum and Mama started work at different times. Sometimes Mum got up early in the morning, gave them breakfast, and then left for work. Sometimes Mama was first downstairs. Sometimes, but not very often, Mum and Mama got up at a reasonable hour and were both around for morning Ablutions and cuddles.

Today was different. Mama had got up early, fed the pups and Dana, and had left for work. She had seemed worried; maybe she was expecting a busy day with her patients (whom Cooper had met when he had visited Mama's work once and found he liked it there because he was able to give Cooper Cuddles to everyone).

Mum hadn't come down by the time Nice Post Lady had delivered her letters. Whisper barked and barked until Nice Post Lady went away. That made

Cooper sad because he usually said "hello" to Nice Post Lady when she brought them letters.

It was at least lunchtime (not that Cooper ever ate lunch but he sometimes cleaned Mum's Yo-Goat bowl for her) when Mum finally shuffled downstairs. Cooper and Whisper went to greet her, their tails wagging. She was still wearing her pyjamas! How unusual!

Her face was pale and she looked tired. Cooper leant against her leg, trying ask what was wrong, but Mum didn't speak Sprockerdor or Woogle, which was a shame because Cooper could have had some very stimulating and educational conversations with her if they all spoke the same language.

Mum went into the kitchen, made a glass of Lup-lup, and then dragged her feet into the living room. Cooper followed close by but made sure not to make Mum trip. He'd done that before and figured if Mum wasn't quite herself the last thing she'd want to do was be accidentally bowled over by an exuberant Sprockerdor.

The glass of Lup-lup wasn't unusual but the lack of Morning Gubble Espresso was. Mum *always* had her Morning Gubble Espresso. This made Cooper more worried than anything else did.

Mum carefully put her Lup-lup on the coffee table before sitting on the sofa. Actually, 'flopping' was a more accurate word, Cooper decided. Mum curled up in the corner of the sofa and pulled the Blankie from the back of it. She wrapped the Blankie around herself and closed her eyes.

Cooper hopped onto the sofa. As always, he put his face right across hers so that she could feel his cheek on her nose, and leant against her shoulder. A full-on Cooper Cuddle.

Mum grumbled something and pushed him away. Then she lay down into the cushions and let out a massive sigh.

Whisper came over too and snuffed Mum's slippered feet. "Goodness Whisper," said Whisper. "Whisper thinks Mum might be Pawly."

"Who's Pauly?" asked Cooper. "Isn't that Granddad?" Mama's daddy was called Paul.

"No, Coop," said Whisper, "Pawly, as in 'not very well'."

"Ooh." Cooper gazed sorrowfully at Mum, who, now that he considered her closely, had a very red nose as well as pale skin and a tired appearance. "Ya, I think you're right."

"Looks like Whisper will have to be Nurse Whisp and make sure Mum is well looked after," said Whisper, clambering onto the sofa as well and lying along Mum's leg. "It's a very Im-paw-tant responsibility." She rested her chin on her paws and let out a sigh almost as massive as Mum's.

Cooper approached Mum once more, anxious not to get too close as Mum clearly didn't want his usual close Cooper Cuddles. "I wonder what *I* could do to make her feel better."

"You could be Carer Coop. Send her Wag, get well soon, thoughts," said Whisper, "and perhaps a gift of some sort." Whisper stretched, letting out a low noise of contentment. "Mum brings Mama gifts when she's Pawly. Maybe Mum would like gifts too."

Now, Cooper was not allowed to pick things up that had not been given to him. Bones were okay, Biz Kits, and the toys Mum and Mama had purchased for both pups – these were fine. But anything else – shoes, pens, iBones, etcetera – these were all off limits. It was one of the first things Cooper had learnt as a baby Sprockerdor.

So Cooper went over to his toy box to have a look for a gift.

Inside his toy box were many things he *was* allowed to pick up, and therefore also deliver to Mum as gifts. So he took Purple Toy, which had three ends and was rubbery, and carried it over to the sofa. He laid it carefully next to Mum's hand, then nuzzled her fingers with his nose.

Mum opened her eyes in a groggy way and smiled at him.

Cooper moved back and sat nicely like a Good Boy. When Mum hadn't noticed Purple Toy, Cooper did a Beg, his paws waving in the air. That usually got Mum's attention.

Mum's smile widened just a smidge but she still ignored Purple Toy and then closed her eyes again.

Cooper went back to the toy box and chose Big Beehive. He placed Big Beehive next to Purple Toy by Mum's hand on the sofa.

Nothing.

He moved back, sat down, and did a Beg. It was a very skilful Beg, one that would definitely make Mum laugh and take notice.

Nothing.

Back to the toy box. He grabbed Small Beehive and lay it next to Big Beehive and Purple Toy.

Nothing.

Mum must be very Pawly to not be responding to any toys and definitely not responding to Cooper doing any Begs. This was rather concerning.

"Mum doesn't seem to be in the mood for gifts," said Cooper, plonking his bottom onto the carpet so he could think properly about the situation.

"Yeah," said Whisper, "she must be very Pawly." Whisper snuggled more firmly into Mum's hip.

"There must be something else I can do," said Cooper. He felt shaky and nervous. Whisper was doing her very responsible job of being Nurse Whisp; now he needed to fulfil his very responsible role of being Carer Coop. He looked around him. The only thing he could see was his long, feathery tail sweeping from side to side in a sort of hopeful way. "I do have a magnificent tail," thought Cooper. "I wonder whether it has magical properties."

He wagged his tail and wag was the same word as Wag, which meant happy. He wanted Mum to feel Wag and by wagging he might just achieve this, in a Magical Wag sense. Magical Wags might work. But if Dana ever heard him utter such a thing she would roll about on the floor like she had when he'd worn his Fleshy Prince boots. She'd call him 'stupid' and 'flaky', although Cooper had never had a flake in his life. He wasn't allowed Choco-lit.

"I won't find out whether it's true unless I try," thought Cooper. He cocked his head until one of his ears fell inside-out and became a puffball on top of his head. Then he prepared himself for action.

He stood cautiously on the sofa next to Mum and did some slow but wide Magical Wags. At least he hoped they were magical. "It must be something one has to do for a long period of time," thought Cooper, so he kept doing it.

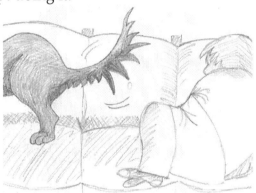

Mum appeared to be snoozing, which was fine. Cooper always felt better after a snooze if he felt Pawly before a snooze.

In the end, Carer Coop lay down near Mum and put his chin on his paws too, just like Nurse Whisp.

And Carer Coop continued to do Magical Wags until he fell asleep.

Afternoon rolled around. The noise of the door opening woke both pups. They ran to the front door to greet Mama, who had returned from work.

Cooper tried to convey how many Magical Wags he had done to help Mum by wiggling his bottom extremely hard. Whisper gave Mama's hand a Lup-lup then returned to the sofa to lie alongside Mum's leg again.

Mum woke too, her hair sticking up as if she'd styled it like a cockatoo, and smiled at Mama as she came into the living room.

Everyone snuggled on the sofa for a while and Carer Coop decided Mum looked a bit better. Her nose was less red and her face was pinker than it had been that morning.

"My Magical Wags worked," thought Cooper. "I shall have to remember that in case anyone else gets Pawly."

Mama gave Carer Coop lots of fusses for looking after Mum.

"I'm an experienced carer now," said Cooper to Whisper. "I should probably complete my nursing degree next so I can go to work with Mum or Mama."

"Whisper thought of doing that once," said Whisper, "but Whisper wasn't able to hold the pen to complete the paperwork."

Cooper rolled onto his back, his paws and feet in the air, and decided it didn't matter. Mama gave him belly rubs and stroked his ears because he was a Good Boy, and that was better payment than any job he could get in the NHS, he reckoned.

CHAPTER 5

Moving Home

Big, brown boxes had begun appearing around their home. Knick-knacks and trinkets and things from the backs of cupboards had been going into the boxes. Mum and Mama filled one box, used sticky tape to keep the lid closed, and then started a new one.

Cooper didn't think much of it until Mama put three of his Blankies into a box and sealed the lid. "Why are my things being put into a box?" asked Cooper.

Whisper did a happy shudder from where she was snoozing on the carpet before lifting her head. "Whatisit?"

"My things." Cooper went over to one of the boxes and put his head into it. It smelled dusty and strange. "Mama put my things into a box."

"Oh yes," said Whisper, "we appear to be moving."

"I'm always moving," said Cooper. "I wag my tail and march around to make sure our home isn't Bungled."

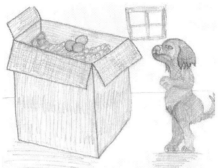

"No," said Whisper with an intelligent air, "we're going to a different home."

"Ooh." Cooper took in the living room. "What's wrong with this one? Is it broken?"

"Whisper doesn't know." Whisper sighed and rolled over on the carpet. She kicked her feet in the air and yawned. "Whisper has moved home several times and each time the home is different. Whisper doesn't notice it being better or worse."

"Ya. Perhaps." Cooper sat very seriously and eyed the boxes. "But why are all our things going into boxes?"

"A van will arrive," said Whisper, "and there will be Lovely Boys to load the boxes into the van. The Lovely Boys will take the boxes into our new home. And we will go in the car, and Mum and Mama will unpack the boxes."

"Ooh." Only three of Cooper's Blankies had gone into the box. That wasn't all of them. Cooper went into his House and dragged his one remaining Blankie through the door after him. Then he went back to the box and dropped his one remaining Blankie into it. "There we go," said Cooper. "That's all of my Blankies."

"S'lovely," said Whisper. "Don't forget your toys."

"Ooh, ya." Cooper padded around the living room, collected his toys one at a time, and placed them into the box. "They are very Im-paw-tant." He cared about his toys a lot. But he cared about his Bally-ballys more than he cared about his other toys. "Oh my goodness! My Bally-ballys!"

"Oh yes," said Whisper. "Mum and Mama might forget the Bally-ballys. Perhaps Cooper had better pack those himself as well."

"But I can't reach my Bally-ballys," said Cooper, his heart falling into his fluffy feet. "They are all in the Walkies bag, and that's hung up higher than I can reach." He sighed forlornly. "I'm a Big Boy but I'm not that big."

"That *is* a predicament," said Whisper, her eyes narrowing in thought. "Whisper's not sure what to suggest."

When Mama came back into the living room, Cooper bounded up to her before sitting down and doing a Beg. His paws flapped in the air a few times as he sat on his back legs.

Mama laughed and looked about her. Was she looking for a toy? That was usually why Cooper did a Beg; he wanted someone to throw a toy for him. But all of Cooper's toys were in the box.

Mama took his Purple Toy out of the box and threw it for him.

Automatically, Cooper pounced on it but then realised what he'd done. "Mama is not making my packing task easy," said Cooper. "She's taking my toys *out* of the box."

"Hoomans are very confusing sometimes," said Whisper.

"Ya." Cooper went into the porch where the Walkies bag was and did a Beg in front of it.

Mama frowned and followed him into the porch. She put her hands on her hips and shook her head. "No," said Mama.

"I know I don't usually have my Bally-ballys when we're not doing Walkies," explained Cooper, "but I would like to pack my Bally-ballys if that's okay, Mama?"

But Mama didn't speak Sprockerdor which was a shame. Stimulating and educational conversations, and all that.

Cooper stomped back into the living room, bowed, huffed, and rolled onto his back with his mouth open.

The cat flap banged and Dana arrived through it, her tail vertical and her head held high. "Hello, stupid puppies."

"Hello, Dana," said Cooper, his voice sorrowful.

"What's the matter with you?" asked Dana. She called him a rude word in Puzzer language as she stalked across the room.

"I'm just sad because we're moving, and my Bally-ballys might be left behind," said Cooper. He rolled back onto his front and rested his chin on his paws.

Dana let out a cruel, teasing laugh. "Stupid puppy. Don't you keep all your possessions safe?" She jumped onto the sofa and curled her fluffy tail around her feet. "I always make sure my Nip is organised and safe just in case I have to move locations at a moment's notice. It's part of the CIA Code of Practise. Don't you do that?"

"No," said Cooper, "I let Mum and Mama look after my Bally-ballys."

"Stupid puppy." And Dana span a few times, then curled up on the sofa to have Sleeps.

Dana had been no help. Cooper felt even worse now he realised he shouldn't have left the responsibility of his Bally-ballys to his parents. That had been a mistake on his part. He puffed out a sigh and wondered helplessly what he could do.

For the next few days, after Cooper had carried home his Bally-bally from Walkies, he refused to let Mama put it back in the Walkies bag. He held onto it tightly and plonked it into the cardboard box with his toys.

But Mama made disgusted noises and gingerly took the Bally-bally back out of the box, holding it with just her thumb and one finger, as if it was covered in poo (it wasn't covered in poo; Cooper checked). Then she threw it back into the Walkies bag.

Cooper's attempts to be responsible for his Bally-ballys were failing. He had a few more stomping, bowing, huffing, and rolling moments but in the end he figured he would just have to accept that some of his Bally-ballys might be left behind.

When moving day arrived, Cooper and Whisper went to Grandma and Granddad's for the afternoon. Dana went too, in her special Cat Carrying Box. Cooper was impressed by the amazing set of impressions Dana was able to do in her Cat Carrying Box. She started with a washing machine, going round and round and making an awful lot of noise. Then she did an impression of a loaf of bread, all bundled up with no feet visible, motionless and silent. Cooper would have given her a round of applause if he'd had hands. He gave her an extra special Wag instead.

Cooper and Whisper weren't allowed on the sofa at Grandma and Granddad's, but Cooper was allowed to lean against Granddad's leg and have an ear fuss, and Whisper and Grandma had girly chats about boys and fashion.

When Mama and Mum came to Grandma and Granddad's to collect them, the sun was dipping low in the sky and Cooper was feeling very sleepy. Mama lifted him into the car (he tried to reason that he could do Walkies to their new home but Mama clearly didn't understand) and they drove away. A moment and a half later, they arrived.

All the furniture from their old home had been taken to their new home which Cooper was pleased about. He and Whisper explored every new room and took in all the Snuffs, of which there were at least seventeen.

Cooper's house was in the kitchen with his bed and Ducky, just like before. His bowls were on the floor, the Biz Kit box he and Whisper shared was on the counter, and their toy box was in the new living room. The Walkies bag was hung up by the back door. Cooper did a Beg just to lift his front half high enough to see inside it. To his surprise and complete relief, he saw that all of his Bally-ballys were present. They *had* been brought from the old home to the new home! He hadn't left any of them behind!

"Oh my Goodness," exclaimed Cooper, whizzing in a circle, "I'm such a Wag Boy."

"Whisper's Wag too," said Whisper, hopping onto the sofa with a groan. "Whisper's had enough of 'get down Whisper' and 'you're not allowed on the sofa, Whisper' at Grandma and Granddad's. Not satisfactory hospitality for a mature Woogle moving home."

Cooper hadn't minded staying on the floor but he knew Whisper was a Woogle of high standards when it came to home comforts.

In any case, it didn't matter. They were at their new home now, his Bally-ballys were all accounted for, and he was feeling rather Wag.

CHAPTER 6

Fwens

Cooper was watching something small and green. The small and green thing was on his Garden Blankie and it looked as if it was sunbathing.

Sunbathing wasn't something that appealed to Cooper, but Whisper loved to do it. She would stretch out on the Garden Blankie and do happy shudders and expose her belly to the sun's warmth. Cooper got very hot in the sun so he mostly stuck to the shade. He was more of a Shade-bather.

Perhaps the small and green thing was called Bertie. Cooper watched as Bertie waddled with his shiny shell over to one side of the Garden Blankie. Then Bertie stopped again. Cooper poked Bertie with his nose. Bertie turned to face Cooper.

"I think we might be Fwens," said Cooper.

Whisper stretched and let out a wide yawn. "Whatisit?"

"Me and Bertie. Fwens."

"S'lovely." Whisper peeked an eye open. "Bertie is a beetle."

"Ooh." Cooper gazed down at his new Fwen. Bertie had such a shiny green shell and round body. Cooper had never seen such a beautiful beetle.

Mum was sunbathing too. She wore sunglasses and had rolled up her trousers to her knees. She had a smiley, smooth look on her face. Mum was definitely a sunbather.

Cooper snuck under her arm and Mum fussed his head. "Hello, Mum," said Cooper, plonking his bottom down.

"Hello, mate," said Mum. At least that's what Cooper imagined she said.

"I have made a Fwen," said Cooper, feeling awfully proud of himself.

Mum continued to fuss his head whilst simultaneously reading her book and expertly sunbathing.

Cooper leant against her side and looked around the garden. He loved their new garden. It had concrete slabs, pebbles to do Wees on, and a big wooden shed to keep his Garden Blankies in. Flouflous grew all over the place in the border, each one a bright shade of grey.

He went to Snuff one large Flou-flou that had long, white petals and a darker middle. "Hello, Fwen Flou-flou."

The Flou-flou swayed about.

Cooper wagged his tail. "I have to name you something as well. It isn't fair for Bertie to have a name and the Flou-flou not to have a name." He stuck his tongue out the side of his mouth and thought very hard. "You look like quite a manly Flou-flou. I shall give you a manly name."

He paced a circle around the garden before he decided.

"Bruce. I shall call you Bruce."

A cackling Cat-cophony sounded from high in a tree. Dana dropped from a branch and landed on all four feet with no issue at all. "Stupid puppy with a stupid name for a flower," laughed Dana.

Cooper pushed out his bottom lip and turned his back on her. "Don't you worry, Bruce," he told the Flou-flou with a tender Snuff, "I think you have a Paw-fect name."

Dana stalked away, still laughing.

Whisper rolled onto her back, her feet and paws sticking up in the air. Her belly expanded and then deflated in a large sigh. She flopped onto her side and fell back to sleep.

Mum sipped her Lup-lup and read her book.

With a flutter of grey wings, a huge bird landed on the fence nearby. Cooper could hardly believe it. Birds almost *never* came into the garden when he was in the garden. Whisper said it was because birds were scared of him. Cooper couldn't work out why. All he wanted to do was be their Fwen.

Whisper lifted her head and ears at the bird.

The bird regarded Cooper with a beady black eye. It made a 'Coop' noise.

"Hello," said Cooper. "I know what you are. You're a Pig Jun."

The Pig Jun cocked its head at him.

"You are rather lovely. I shall call you Pablo."

"Aww," said Whisper, "Pablo the Pig Jun."

"Ya. It's a lovely name for a lovely bird."

Pablo seemed to agree. He puffed up his feathers and strutted up and down the fence. "Coop, Cooooop," said Pablo. He pecked at the wood of the fence, perhaps to eat a beetle or two.

Cooper was pleased Pablo knew his name, but hoped Bertie wouldn't fall foul to Pablo's appetite.

Another small crawly thing scuttled about next to the Garden Blankie. It was different from Bertie—it was dark brown and had three tiny parts to its body. It had lots of legs, more than Cooper but less than the spider Cooper had seen on the ceiling, the one that Mum had sucked up with the Nemesis whilst doing housework. Cooper instantly loved the small crawly thing because it was teeny-tiny and brown and scuttled so wonderfully.

The small crawly thing stopped by Cooper's paw.

"Hello, small crawly thing," said Cooper.

"That's an ant," said Whisper.

"Ooh. S'lovely." Cooper put his chin on his paws so that his nose was very close to the ant. "Hello, small crawly ant."

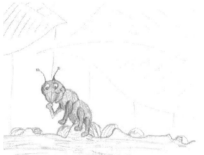

The ant scurried about, clearly going about some very Im-paw-tant business.

"His name is Anthony," Cooper told Whisper, "and he is most definitely my best Fwen."

"I thought Rocket was your best Fwen," said Whisper.

"Perhaps Anthony can be my second-best Fwen," said Cooper.

Whisper snored as she fell back to sleep.

"Hello, Anthony."

For a long time, Cooper conversed with Anthony about Im-paw-tant issues as well as day-to-day subjects.

"Did you know," said Cooper to Whisper, "because of the Dam Pendic, the National Health Motorway Services are in desperate need of Anty Bodies? And Anthony and his friends are off on a journey to donate their Anty Bodies to science to battle the Dam Pendic."

Whisper slept on.

"Well, I think it's very serious and Im-paw-tant." Cooper put his chin back atop his paws and gazed proudly at his new second-best Fwen, Anthony.

Anthony was brown, just like Cooper. But he was also different in a lot of ways. He was teeny-tiny, had two extra legs, and no tail. Differences, Cooper decided, were a good thing.

After lunch, it was time for some Walkies. Whisper stayed at home due to her Old Lady Legs, which meant Cooper got Mum all to himself. Cooper was teaching Mum that walking more quickly was preferable to walking as a steady pace. He wanted to get to the park as fast as possible. He tugged and pulled on his lead with all his might.

Mum didn't seem to understand this training which was unusual as Cooper assumed Mum was fairly intelligent. She kept making him walk in a backwardly direction, which was very annoying.

When they *finally* got to the park, Cooper saw something that made his heart leap as high as Dana hopping over the Puppy-gate. A tall, black Gorgeous Lad with floppy ears was trotting about on the grass.

Cooper waited until Mum unclipped his lead and scrambled over to the Gorgeous Lad. "Hello, Rocket," he said. He was breathless, both from running and his excitement.

"Hello, Coop, mate," Rocket said, his tail wagging. "Not seen you in a while."

"Ya. We have had Walkies in other areas. But I'm very happy to see you." Cooper rolled onto his back in front of Rocket just to prove this.

Rocket Snuffed Cooper's bottom with interest. "I see you've had beef and vegetables for breakfast. Wet Kibble! You are lucky!"

"Ya. Mum and Mama discovered something very interesting. If they give me and Whisp some Wet Kibble, I will eat my Krunchy Kibble more quickly."

"Funny how that turned out," said Rocket with an air of amusement.

"Ya, I won't ever eat Krunchy Kibble quickly again. That way we will always have Wet Kibble."

Uncle Matthew, who was Rocket's Hooman Daddy, and Mum walked together (although at a distance because of the Dam Pendic), and Uncle Matthew threw a Bally-bally for Cooper and Rocket to chase.

Cooper's skills were much Poo-perior when it came to Retrieval Services. He let Rocket catch the Bally-bally sometimes, to make it fair.

Rocket dropped the Bally-bally with a disgusted look. "This Bally-bally is covered in mud," he said.

"Ooh," said Cooper, "is that not a good thing?" Cooper thought back to his experiences with mud and decided he liked the stuff. It made light-coloured dogs look very beautiful when they were covered in it. It was his life's work to make all light-coloured dogs brown with mud.

"I don't like it at all. It's dirty and makes other things dirty with its presence." Rocket stared down sorrowfully at the Bally-bally Cooper had just let him catch. "But mud is at least better than sand." He shook his head so that his ears flapped about. "Sand is out to get me. It simply won't leave me alone when I'm on the beach."

But Cooper liked sand as well. It felt nice between his toes and was very sandy. He and Rocket were different in that respect.

"I have to wash the Bally-bally in the sea when it gets covered in sand," said Rocket. "I prefer my Bally-ballys clean and tidy."

Cooper supposed they could compromise. He didn't care about a clean Bally-bally but it was obviously Im-paw-tant to Rocket. And Cooper loved Rocket. "We shall have to wash our Bally-bally in the pond," said Cooper.

So in they went. At first, Cooper was careful where he put his paws because of his previous Pawly paw incident. But soon, splashes happened all around them which caused both Mum and Uncle Matthew to shout. In the end, Mum and Uncle Matthew stopped shouting and they all had a lovely time in, or near, the pond.

Once Cooper and Rocket were out of Beans, they stepped out of the pond and had some good Shakes.

"Are you happy now that the Bally-bally is clean?" asked Cooper hopefully.

"Yes," replied Rocket. "The pond is a great way to wash a Bally-bally."

Cooper agreed but still didn't understand why Rocket didn't like mud or sand. "I suppose," he thought, "it's good that we are different. If all my Fwens liked all the same things as me, life would be awfully boring."

CHAPTER 7

A Sprockerdor Spruce

As the weather got warmer, summer shone wonderfully down on Whisper in the garden. Cooper didn't seem to like the hot weather. "Of course," thought Whisper, "he *is* a Sprockerdor and not good at sunbathing, but Whisper has absolutely no idea why he is panting and looking grumpy."

"I'm too hot," said Cooper with his tongue lolling out. "My dark, thick fur makes it hard to stay cool."

Whisper couldn't think why he'd *want* to stay cool when it was so Wag in the sun but she gave him a sympathetic look because he really did look unhappy.

The next day, Mum led him into the kitchen and got out some scissors and a buzzy thing that made some of his hair fall off. She clipped his legs and his tummy, trimmed his ears and the fluff between his fingers and toes. This meant that some parts of Cooper were not so hot anymore, and he seemed happier. He looked a bit less fluffy but still had patches of fluff here and there.

But his fur just kept growing back. It was as if someone had put fertiliser on some dark brown grass and watered the dark brown grass thoroughly until it grew as tall as the trees. At least, that's what Whisper imagined it was like.

Once the Dam Pendic was over, and professionals were allowed to make pups beautiful again, Mum took Cooper to a Local Lady Professional.

Whisper waved them off at the door and went to have Sleeps in peace.

It was Friday afternoon, so Dana was out preparing for Nip Night with her fellow Puzzer cats. Apparently there were Im-paw-tant things to purchase for the weekly festivities. Whisper wasn't entirely sure what Nip Night entailed, but Dana always came back the morning after looking fairly worse for wear.

Amid a dream about Biz Kits and naughty squirrels, Whisper was woken by a paw that seemed a lot less fluffy than the one she was used to.

"Whisp?" said Cooper, prodding her with his newly unfluffy paw. "Are you having Sleeps?"

"Yeah," said Whisper, stretching. When she opened her eyes and caught sight of him, she immediately stood. "Why, Coop! Where has all your fluff gone?"

"I had a Spruce from the nice Local Lady Professional," said Cooper, sitting up straight with a proud look in his eye. "She cleaned my ears and de-fluffed my paws and made my tummy and legs all neat. And then, because I was a Very Good Boy and we were done early, she threw a Bally-bally in her garden for me. It was so lovely!"

"What is *that*?" asked Whisper, pushing her nose under his chin to Snuff something attached to his collar.

"Ooh, ya, that's the bowtie she gave me. I love it *so* much."

Whisper frowned. What service Cooper had experienced! And how handsome and neat he looked now!

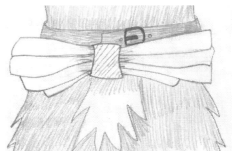

"Well," said Whisper, "Whisper will definitely have to ask Mum if she can have her own Spruce with the Local Lady Professional. Whisper could do with a new style. Perhaps a highlight or two, or train-tracks." Whisper wasn't sure what train-tracks were, but she liked trains and tracking things with her nose. So they must be the height of fashion.

"Ooh ya. I mean," said Cooper lowering his head a little, "you look beautiful as you are, but maybe you could look even *more* beautiful if you went to see the Local Lady Professional."

It was settled then—Whisper would have to convince Mum and Mama she was simply too hot, and that her fur was not neat enough, and then they would take her to the Local Lady Professional who made pups beautiful.

So the next day, whilst on Walkies, Whisper rolled in as much fox and badger perfume as she could and then waded into the pond, making her legs smell of the green weed that grew there. She lay in the muddiest areas she could find and panted her best ever hot pants, even though she wasn't that hot. She rubbed against every tree to make her coat stand up on end in patches, and did Shakes so that Mum and Mama would think she had dirty, itchy ears.

On the way home, Whisper plotted her make-over, feeling rather pleased with herself that she'd managed to do so much excellent convincing. She was sure to get a Spruce with the Local Lady Professional now.

The minute they arrived home, Mama got out the hose.

The hose was not Whisper's Fwen. It was possibly less of a Fwen to Whisper than the Nemesis, which sucked up all the dirt and insects from the carpet and made Whisper run away. The hose squirted cold water whenever Mum or Mama turned the big tap on the wall it was connected to. It gave Dreaded Washes to dirty pups.

Mama held Whisper steady and directed the hose at her sticking-up fur.

Whisper closed her eyes as her spirits fell. She was getting Dreaded Washes. That meant Shampoop and freezing water and Scrubby-scrubs. Whisper braced herself; she couldn't get away because Mama was a lot stronger than her.

Whilst Whisper got Dreaded Washes, the smell of Shampoop wafting into her nose, jealously flooded every part of her. It was *so* unfair that Cooper got to go to the nice Local Lady Professional and had come back looking so gorgeous. Whisper had done her best to convince Mum and Mama she needed a Spruce too, but it had all been for nothing.

Instead of getting a womanly bowtie on her collar, she was getting cold, horrible Dreaded Washes. It was absolutely not Wag.

Later, when she was nearly dry and wrapped in a towel on the bed in the kitchen, Mama gave her a sorry look and offered her a Biz Kit. Whisper couldn't deny herself a Biz Kit—she'd done plenty of exercise and had had Dreaded Washes, she deserved it—but refused to wag her tail. She put her head under the towel and sulked.

Cooper's warm weight rested against her side. "Are you okay, Whisp?"

"Whisper's upset," said Whisper. "Whisper tried as hard as Whisper could to convince Mum and Mama she required a Spruce from the Local Lady Professional, but instead, Whisper got Dreaded Washes. Which is less than satisfactory." She kept her head under the towel.

"I'm sorry, Whisp," said Cooper, "I suppose because Sprockerdors have longer fur than Woogles,

Woogles aren't that difficult to maintain and don't need a Spruce."

Whisper didn't reply. She just let out a massive sigh, blowing the edge of the towel so it fluttered.

"Which is rather lovely, I think." Cooper's voice held a smile. "Like I said, you're so beautiful already that you don't need a Spruce like Cooper does. You're perfect just as you are."

"But Whisper didn't get a bowtie," said Whisper in a final attempt at being jealous.

"Local Lady Professional said I will need to go again for a Spruce soon," said Cooper. "I like the bowtie I've got now and intend to wear it forever. If she gives me another bowtie next time I go, I shall give it to you as a brotherly gift."

Whisper poked her head out of the towel. "Cooper would?"

Cooper blinked down at her. "Ya. Because you're my sister and I love you."

"Aww. Whisper loves Coop too, Coop." Whisper snuggled up to his side.

Even if Whisper didn't get a Spruce every now and again, at least she had the best brother ever. Hopefully it wouldn't be long until he next needed a Spruce, and if the weeks passed and Mum didn't take him to the Local Lady Professional, Whisper would just have to speed things along a bit. She knew where a fine area of fox perfume was, and was sure she could teach Cooper how to roll in it.

CHAPTER 8

Stealing Sausages

Dana was a trained assassin with the CIA. She was highly qualified in planting bombs, napalm, poisoning her enemies, and Paw-smacking.

The Paw-smacking qualification came in very handy with the Stupid Puppies. Whisper wasn't so annoying these days, but when Dana had first been brought home, she'd spent a good six weeks doing some excellent Paw-smacking on Whisper's nose.

The young pup Cooper was another matter. He wasn't quite sure of the way that things were done yet. He wasn't aware that everything Dana said was fact, that she was the authority on everything and everyone, and only her Hooman Slaves, Mum and Mama, stood in her way to World Domination.

So, more Paw-smacks were definitely in order. Dana carried these out whenever she felt it appropriate.

Summer was Dana's favourite season. She liked to roll on the grass in the warmth of the sun, stretch her fingers and toes out, and recharge her batteries. She was practising for when she no longer needed Mum and Mama to feed her Puzzer cat Kibble, that hopeful time in the future when her CIA superiors would install the solar panel and she would become a Cyborg Registered Agent Puzzer.

That day was far away, but Dana didn't care. It would arrive and then her plans would come to fruition.

A wide yawn caught her unawares and Dana jumped when a loud scraping sound filled the garden. She looked over to where the sound had come from.

Mum was in the shed, wrestling with a contraption she hadn't taken out for a whole year.

Memories flashed across Dana's mind—sweet and succulent smells, tasty titbits, and a big, hot appliance that she was not allowed to get close to.

Barbecue.

Mum pulled the barbecue over to the patio and went back into the shed to get a bag of something heavy. Black, shiny, pebble type things tumbled into the bowl area of the barbecue with a clatter. Then Mum pushed some white sticks under the pebble type things. She lit a match.

After getting up from her warm, grassy spot, Dana padded over. Her whiskers fluttered as she took in the chemical smells and then the scent of smoke. Fire? Was Mum trying to set the garden alight?

Excellent. Dana did love a bit of destruction.

But, no, the only things on fire were the black pebble type things.

Shame.

Dana's sun-addled mind nudged her to remember the meat, the dripping juices, and the wonderful smells. Her mouth watered.

She snorted in disgust at herself. She was a trained assassin. She didn't succumb to bodily needs, like hunger, and especially not when there wasn't even any food nearby.

"What's that?" The loud and frankly irritating, Stupid Puppy voice made Dana's ears hurt.

She turned slowly towards Cooper and rolled her eyes. "That is the barbecue. Mum is preparing it for food heating and deliciousness."

"Ooh." Cooper's bottom plonked onto the patio. "Are we allowed the food or will Mum and Mama be eating it?"

"Stupid puppy," said Dana. "Do you think I've asked them? I do not concern myself with such matters."

Cooper sighed miserably and hung his head. "I'm sorry, Dana. I did not know you did not know the situation." He cocked his head one way, then the other. "I assumed you knew because you are very wise."

"I am," said Dana, a flick of her tail displaying her annoyance.

She took a moment to gather her thoughts. It *was* a lovely day and later promised delicious food. It was ever-so tiring to be constantly evil to the siblings she happened to live with (through no choice of her own). Perhaps she could be, if not kind, civil to the frankly annoying puppy and his big stripy sister.

"Sometimes," said Dana careful to keep an element of disgust in her voice, "Mum and Mama give us small morsels of food when they have a barbecue. And the food is high quality, very scrumptious. I suggest you act like a Very Good Boy and then you may receive such treats."

"Ooh," said Cooper, wondrously, "I shall! I shall!" He bounded about a bit with his huge paws and feathery tail.

Dana chose not to laugh at his antics. She didn't want to appear too kind, and it was best he was not encouraged anyway.

Smoke began to curl upwards from the barbecue. Orange flames licked the black, pebble type things. Mum used a metal rod to poke them, which made more flames and more smoke. She coughed and backed away.

"Oh, Whisper's Goodness," said Whisper, who had just stepped out of the house and into the garden. "Does Mum need medical attention? Must Whisper be Nurse Whisp?"

But Mum stopped coughing. She went over to Whisper first to fuss her ears, then to Cooper, who wagged his tail brightly. When she came over to Dana, Dana regrettably allowed Mum to fuss her ears too, always keeping in mind the meat she may receive as a result.

Whisper and Cooper exchanged a meaningful glance.

Dana stuck her tail into the air and sauntered off. She didn't care that the Stupid Puppies thought she was soft. If she behaved in a soft and affectionate way, she was more likely to receive a sausage or similar from the barbecue.

Dana took up residence on the branch of her favourite tree at the edge of the garden. She watched as the flames of the barbecue shrunk to nothing, leaving only glowing embers. Mum and Mama brought out three plates, three glasses for Lup-lup, and three sets of cutlery, and put them on the garden table.

Dana had the training and CIA education to recognise that three sets of dinner items meant that another Hooman would be joining them. She hoped it would be Grandpa because he might be wearing his yellow jumper which Dana very much enjoyed kneading. But Grandpa always came with Granny because he needed help getting around. And Grandpa and Granny would definitely mean four sets of dinner items rather than three. It could be a different member of the Hooman family, but most of them came in pairs as well.

When the sun was halfway down the sky, indicating nearly Din-dins time, there was a knock at the gate. The Stupid Puppies went to see who it was, so Dana jumped down from the tree and made out she wasn't bothered. She kept one eye on the gate, however, just in case the identity of the visitor was important.

It was Auntie Carol, who lived next door with her two Hooman boys and often looked after Dana if Mum, Mama, and the Stupid Puppies went on Holly Bobs.

Dana pricked up her ears. Out of all the candidates Dana could come up with, Auntie Carol was by far the best. Sometimes, Dana went round Auntie Carol's home when she was sick of the Stupid Puppies, and they watched intellectual programmes on the Velly Tision. Dana particularly enjoyed 'Gogglebox' which was a highly artistic and scientific study of Hooman interaction.

Auntie Carol fussed the Stupid Puppies first—of course, they always got preference and one day Dana would make them pay—and then came over to Dana.

Dana did her very skilled impression of a tiny Puzzer cat in need of love and affection. She made her eyes big, rubbed her whole body against Auntie Carol's legs, and did some very pretty meows.

Auntie Carol was fooled once again. She gave Dana many smooths and fusses and talked to her in a silky voice.

Dana laughed inwardly. She was definitely in for some kind of meaty barbecue reward from this one.

The Hoomans sat on the garden chairs and drank bubbly Lup-lup poured from a bottle. The Stupid Puppies milled around their legs, hankering for fusses or similar. Dana turned her nose up at this. She had received her fuss and now simply needed to wait until the food was ready.

Mum brought out a large platter of raw meat. Dana would have happily eaten the whole lot as it was, but Hoomans seemed obsessed with cooking their meat, so she allowed this, curling up beside Auntie Carol's chair to wait.

At several moments, the smells of cooking meat were almost unbearable. Dana's mouth watered, much to her annoyance, and the Stupid Puppies seemed to be fairing no better. A thin string of spit hung down from the side of Whisper's mouth, and Cooper's eyes were fixed on the barbecue as if by hypnosis.

Finally, Mum took the fizzling, sizzling meat from the barbecue and placed an equal amount on each of the three plates.

Dana's stomach fell. Where were her tasty treats? She'd been such a loving and affectionate cat! How dare the Hoomans deprive her of such wonderful morsels! Perhaps Auntie Carol would give her something off her plate.

As the three Hoomans ate, Dana attempted several times to get Auntie Carol's attention. She jumped into her lap, stood on her back legs with her paws on the chair and gave Auntie Carol head buts, and did some pretty meows.

But Auntie Carol either ignored her, put her back on the floor, or frowned at her. What was wrong with her? Didn't Auntie Carol know Dana was due some meat?

Dana would simply have to use her CIA skills to steal something from Auntie Carol's plate. So, she crouched under Mum's chair where she could stay hidden. She waited, waited, and then waited some more.

Finally, Auntie Carol stood, having only half finished her Din-dins.

This was Dana's chance! She waited until Auntie Carol had walked halfway to the house, until she was far enough away to not be able to save her Din-dins. Then Dana darted out from under the chair, jumped neatly onto the table top, and grabbed a sausage in her mouth.

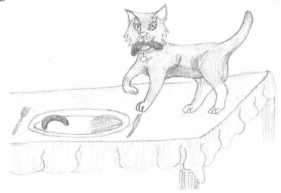

Shouting began—Dana had expected this. But she had the perfect place to hide with her prize.

She ran across the garden, hopped over the gate, and crawled under Mum's car.

At last! The delicious morsel she had worked so hard for was hers! She almost shouted "mine, all mine!" but that would have given her hiding place away.

The shouting died down after a few seconds, which was preferable. Dana required peace and quiet to eat, especially when the food she was eating smelled so delicious.

Once the sausage was all gone, and her paws and face were clean, Dana stretched out under the car and sighed. Stupid Hoomans leaving their Din-dins unattended. Stupid Puppies for not thinking of a way to steal the food they so desperately craved.

She, Dana, was top animal; she was the superior being in the house. No one else matched her intelligence, her skill, or her cunning.

Once she'd had a little sleep and had woken up cold from being under the shady car, Dana strolled back into the garden to recharge in the sun.

Mum, Mama, and Auntie Carol were sitting on the garden chairs, drinking their bubbly Lup-lup, and smiling. Clearly none of them were too concerned about Dana's stealthy stealing of the scrumptious sausage.

Whisper and Cooper were lying down now. They were clearly out of Beans after all the excitement of Auntie Carol being there and Bally-ballys being thrown for them, and their boring, stale-tasting Kibble.

"Evening, Stupid Puppies," said Dana, stalking a path in front of them.

"Hello, Dana," said Whisper, rolling onto her side in the fading sunshine.

"Did you enjoy your sausage?" asked Cooper. For some reason, there was an amused twinkle in his eye.

Dana narrowed her eyes at him. "It was satisfactory. Not the best sausage I've eaten but certainly worth the hassle of obtaining it." She wanted to gloat more, to parade her death-defying feat in their faces but she didn't want to look stuck-up.

81

"And it tasted meaty, did it?" asked Cooper, the twinkle in his eye growing.

"Of course. What else would it taste like? Stupid Puppy."

"Oh maybe," said Whisper as she lifted her head, "Whisper reckons it would have probably tasted like some kind of meat substitute."

"Why would it do that?" asked Dana loudly, fiercely.

"Because," said Cooper, "Auntie Carol is a vegetarian. She doesn't eat meat at all."

"So," said Whisper, "the sausage you ate had no pork, beef, chicken, or lamb in it."

"No meat?" screamed Dana, jumping about a foot off the ground. "How dare she have non-meat sausages on her plate for me to steal! Absolutely terrible! The mere suggestion!"

Cooper and Whisper laughed gently. "Don't worry, Dana," said Cooper, "I bet it still tasted lovely, didn't it?"

"No!" Dana scampered over to her tree and climbed it, hiding her sorry self away in the branches. If she hadn't had fur, her face would have been bright red.

How embarrassing! Fancy being duped into stealing something that didn't even have meat in it! She would have to get revenge on Auntie Carol for this misdemeanour. Auntie Carol would pay!

As her tummy gurgled happily, so full of the sausage she refused to admit had been most scrumptious, she dug her claws into the branch of the tree and imagined all the ways she could cause these Hoomans, and their Stupid Puppy accomplices, to be eradicated.

CHAPTER 9

Old Lady Legs

After Dana's sausage shenanigans, Whisper and Cooper got substantially more treats than usual. Whisper thought this might be because Mum and Mama felt sorry for them—after all, they hadn't had sausages at the barbecue, but Dana had, and that had been rather unfair.

After a few weeks of many Biz Kits, pieces of delicious cheese, and slices of scrumptious ham, Whisper noticed Cooper's belly had become rounder.

"Coop," said Whisper one day after Din-dins, "Whisper reckons you're looking a bit Tumbly."

"Tumbly?" asked Cooper. "Ooh. I suppose I had better start watching my weight." He looked more closely at Whisper. "You know what, Whisp? You're looking a bit Tumbly yourself."

"Is Whisper?" Whisper tried to look at her own belly but the angle was awkward and she ended up with her head upside-down between her elbows. "Maybe Whisper should think about doing some star jumps or something."

"Ya," said Cooper, "I can help you with that. I'm very good at encouraging other dogs to run around."

"Run away," corrected Whisper.

Cooper apparently didn't hear her.

So that afternoon, when Mama took them both to their favourite Walkies field, Whisper and Cooper ran around a lot more than usual. They chased one another, had Plays where they tried to chew one another's feet, and scampered after the Bally-bally when Mama threw it.

By the time they got home, Whisper was thoroughly out of Beans. She flopped onto her back on the sofa and fell straight to sleep. Even the smells of Mama cooking Mama and Mum's Din-dins didn't make her lift her head.

Later, when it was time for Evening Ablutions, Mama beckoned for Whisper to get down from the sofa and go outside. Whisper groaned low in her throat and inched off the sofa one leg at a time. To her dismay, her back legs had gone completely stiff and could barely hold her weight.

Her bottom sunk onto the carpet, with her front half following close behind.

Mama frowned and sat next to her on the carpet. She ruffled Whisper's ears and stroked her back, talking in calming tones. Then she spoke to Mum worriedly.

Whisper tried again to get up but everything seemed glued to the carpet. "Oh Coop," said Whisper, "Whisper's got an issue,"

"Oh no," said Cooper. "What's the matter?"

"Well, perhaps it's two issues," said Whisper, trying to inspect her own back legs. "One issue is Whisper's right leg, and the other issue is Whisper's left leg."

"What a predicament," said Cooper coming over to nudge his head against Mama's cheek. He looked down at Whisper with concern. "I'm sure Mum will fix your legs though. She fixed my paw when my paw was Pawly."

"Whisper reckons Whisper's Old Lady Legs must be Pawly too," said Whisper. Her hips ached and her legs didn't seem to be doing what she wanted them to.

In the end, Mum and Mama lifted Whisper around the middle until she could stand. They had to hold onto her as she walked out into the garden and had some wobbly Wees in the grass. Then they helped her back inside.

Once Whisper was on the dog bed ready for Sleeps, she felt much more Wag. Perhaps her Pawly Old Lady Legs would get better in a minute. Maybe it was only temporary.

Mum got her Din-dins bowl and tipped a small amount of Krunchy Kibble in it. Then she took a purple box from the cupboard and pulled a bottle out of it. She measured out some liquid from the bottle and squirted it into Whisper's Din-dins bowl.

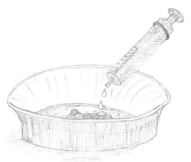

The bowl hit the floor with a soft clang. Automatically, Whisper ate the small amount of Krunchy Kibble that was covered in the liquid. It tasted like Krunchy Kibble so Whisper wasn't too bothered about the liquid. In fact, she cleaned the liquid that had fallen off the Krunchy Kibble from the Din-dins bowl until it shone.

"That looks like the Metty Cam I had when I went to have my Special Puperation," said Cooper. "You know, when they removed bits from my manly area to stop me accidentally becoming a daddy."

"Goodness," said Whisper, "Whisper had a similar procedure when Whisper was a lot less mature." She wracked her three brain cells (including the two in her tail) to remember whether she'd had a similar liquid then. She decided that she had.

"It'll make it all better then," said Cooper. "When I had my Special Puperation, I felt very sore in my manly area. But once I'd had the Metty Cam, I felt much better." He gazed down solemnly at Whisper's back legs. "I hope it makes you feel less sore, Whisp."

"Yeah, so does Whisper," said Whisper. She stretched on the dog bed, all her muscles and joints creaking and aching, until she was as comfy as she could make herself.

Cooper snuggled up to her side, a warm, lumpy weight against her, and snuffed her ears. He gave her left ear an affectionate lick. "And you tell me if you need anything in the night. I can be Carer Coop for you."

"Thanks, Coop," said Whisper, her eyes starting to droop.

As Mum and Mama walked upstairs and the kitchen was left in silence apart from Cooper's little sighs of worry, Whisper felt herself dropping into some serious, deep Sleeps.

In the morning, Cooper was on his feet the moment footsteps could be heard from upstairs. If Mum and Mama were up and about, that meant Breakfast Kibble and Morning Ablutions would be happening soon.

Whisper didn't want to jump straight up like Cooper had. She stayed lying down but put up her head and ears, and wagged her tail when Mum and Mama arrived downstairs.

Mama came over to Whisper and stroked her head in a calm way.

That was nice because Whisper's insides were buzzing about like bees around a Flou-flou. What if she couldn't stand up? What if she had to do her Morning Ablutions on the bed because she was desperate and couldn't get up to go outside? What if Mum and Mama decided she was too much of an Old Lady to be allowed to live with them? Would she have to go to an Old Woogle's Home?

Mama gave her lots of reassuring rubs and strokes and fusses around her hips and back legs, which seemed to warm up Whisper's muscles and joints.

It was time to attempt to stand.

This time Mama just coaxed Whisper with her voice rather than using her hands to help Whisper up. And by some amazing luck, Whisper's legs and hips and muscles and joints all did what they were supposed to do. She was able to lift each foot, and each paw, without anything hurting and without anything behaving as if it was Pawly. She even did a big, long stretch that made her point her toes and reach forwards with her paws as far as she could. It felt good to stretch everything out.

All four legs held her upright with minimal effort, and Whisper wagged her tail more enthusiastically.

Cooper began to hop around, clearly thrilled that Whisper's Old Lady Legs were showing no ill effects from the day before.

"Whisper's vertical," said Whisper with a similar level of thrill, "and Whisper's ready for another long Walkies!"

Cooper stopped hopping around and looked at her very seriously. "I think you should take it easy," said Cooper, "at least until you've rested a bit longer." He grimaced. "I think the long Walkies did you in yesterday."

Mum and Mama seemed to think the same. After breakfast and Morning Ablutions (which Whisper completed with top marks and no aches or wobbles), Whisper was led to the sofa and given a Biz Kit. Mama sat with her and gave her fusses as Mum busied herself putting Poopy-bags and Bally-ballys into her coat pockets.

Cooper knew what this meant. He jumped around as if he had springs in his feet and got royally told off by Mum when he got in the way.

Whisper watched sorrowfully as Mum attached Cooper's lead to his collar and led him outside. They disappeared through the gate for Walkies.

After letting out a huge sigh, Whisper looked up at Mama. "Well, there you go," said Whisper, "Whisper supposes Whisper needs to resign to the fact that Whisper will be unable to have long or energetic Walkies for the foreseeable future."

Mama ruffled her ears and scratched Whisper's belly. Whisper thought she felt sympathy through Mama's hand.

"Perhaps, once Whisper has had a small rest, Whisper will be able to resume normal activities once more."

Mama appeared to agree with that. She hugged Whisper and kissed the top of her head.

Whisper did another sigh, then wiggled her bottom until it was wedged into Mama's side. She leaned back and grinned at Mama, her tongue hanging out.

"Good girl," said Mama—these were words Whisper understood in Hooman language.

"Oh, Whisper is," said Whisper. It was better to take it easy for now than to have to go into an Old

Woogle's Home and have morning Ablutions on the bed because her Old Lady Legs weren't doing the things they were asked. She could cope with short Walkies and days on the sofa if it meant she could stay with Mama and Mum and Cooper and Dana.

CHAPTER 10

Rock Pools

For the second time in Cooper's life, his Bally-ballys, Blankies, and toys were being packed up. This time, rather than a box being the desired container, they were going into a large bag with a zip.

He watched as Mum packed more of his belongings, as well as spare bowls and leads, into the bag, with his head on one side.

Whisper slid herself off the sofa and stretched her Old Lady Legs. "Cooper has a very confused look on Cooper's face," said Whisper before letting out a large yawn.

"I *am* confused," said Cooper. "My things are being packed again. Are we moving home *again*?" He looked around. "This home works very well for me; I'm not sure I want to move."

"No," said Whisper, "Whisper and Cooper and Mum and Mama are going on Holly Bobs."

"What's Holly Bobs?" asked Cooper.

"It's a relaxing few days where the family goes in the car and stays somewhere for Sleeps. Walkies will be had, ones Whisper and Cooper haven't been on before, and there may be Chiplets."

"Ooh," said Cooper. His mouth watered at the thought of Chiplets but a moment later his eyes went wide. "Not in the car, though!"

"Yes, in the car," said Whisper.

"Ooh. I don't like the car." Cooper sighed. "Maybe Mum and Mama will let me do Walkies to the Holly Bobs place. Ya, I think that will be better."

But the next day Cooper was made to jump into the boot with Whisper, and Mum and Mama got into the front.

Cooper watched the world go by out of the back window, his nose making mucky stains on the glass. The car rumbled along roads and motorways and earthy paths for a long time. Whisper lay down on the floor of the boot to have some Sleeps. Jealousy flashed through Cooper because he wished he could be as relaxed as Whisper always was in the car.

Eventually, they arrived at a small cottage. The first thing that hit Cooper's nose was a salty, fishy smell. It was similar to a Snuff he associated with Walkies on the beach which he found very Wag. The beach was a place to have Plays and have Bally-ballys thrown during Retrieval Services.

"Oh, Whisp," said Cooper, enthralled, "I think I love Holly Bobs already."

"Yeah," said Whisper, "Holly Bobs is almost as Wag as Biz Kits."

After Mum and Mama got all their belongings into the cottage, Cooper and Whisper spent many minutes Snuffing the floors, the walls, the furniture, and anything else they could get their noses into. Cooper detected the sea, some sand, and various foods he probably wasn't allowed, as well as some that he hopefully was allowed. He also recognised the Snuffs of other pups. Had other people stayed in the Holly Bobs cottage before them?

Mama took them both for Walkies through some fields, with Cooper completing sufficient Retrieval Services to make him out of breath.

When they got back, Mum had organised all their belongings around the cottage and had filled a bowl with cold Lup-lup ready for their return.

"This cottage Snuffs of so many nice things," said Cooper as he and Whisper stretched out on the rug, out of Beans from their Bally-bally-related activities.

"Yeah," said Whisper, who'd done less running about than Cooper on Walkies but still appeared out of Beans. "S'lovely. Sufficiently comfortable and cosy."

The afternoon was spent lazing about whilst Mum and Mama went out, then they came back and a man delivered a pizza. Cooper and Whisper were given a small piece of Krunchy Krust as a post-Din-dins snack.

That night, Cooper slept in the fabric travel House and Whisper slept on a bed on the floor, covered in a special Holly Bobs Blankie. In the morning, they all had breakfast together.

"When do you think we will have Chiplets?" asked Cooper.

Whisper shuttered her eyes in thought. "Whisper reckons at some point during the Holly Bobs. Usually if we sit at a table outside, and Mum and Mama order Chiplets as *their* food, Whisp and Coops might have Chiplets then."

"It doesn't give me a lot of time to prepare myself," said Cooper with a frown. "What if I don't feel like Chiplets at the time we are offered them?"

"Whisper always feels like Chiplets," said Whisper. "And usually three are presented to Whisper for munching."

"Ya," said Cooper, brightening a bit, "Chiplets are an all-day-any-place type of food, aren't they?"

Whisper simply nodded.

Another trip in the car and they arrived at a place similar to the beach near where they lived. It Snuffed more strongly of sand and salt and fish than their Holly Bobs cottage. Small Hoomans ran about with huge Bally-ballys that made Cooper's own Bally-ballys look like pieces of Krunchy Kibble in comparison, and gulls screeched overhead.

The day's Walkies were taken up and down the beach, with much Retrieval Services, although Whisper was forced to remain on the lead the whole time. "Whisper's got an issue with Foot-bally-ballys," said Whisper, looking guilty. "Once, Mum had to pay a man to replace one that Whisper had accidentally popped."

"Ooh goodness," said Cooper, imagining the devastation.

On the way back, then went closer to the water, near some rocks. Cooper scampered up one of the rocks, his feet slipping on the wet surface. His heart beat faster as he climbed higher and higher, until he came to a gap between two big rocks.

In the gap was a small pool of Lup-lup. Cooper did a special-excited bark to let Mama and Mum know where he was and also to tell them he had found something special-exciting. Mama climbed up after him and used a happy voice to say his name.

Cooper wagged his tail and looked down into the pool of Lup-lup. He bent his head and Lup-lupped some of it, but shook his head when it tasted horrible. "No," Mama said and he decided he agreed with her.

He gazed into the pool between the rocks, interested in the contents. Was there pirate treasure in there? Food, perhaps? Could he see any Fwens?

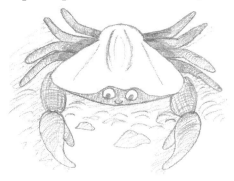

An orange beetle-like thing with big claws on the front and a wide shell scuttled sideways out of some seaweed. Cooper yapped at it and it scowled at him, sinking back into the pool between the rocks.

A flutter-splash of movement caught his eye. A small, silver fish was flicking about near the top of the Lup-lup. Cooper poked it with his nose, which tickled. The fish swam away and disappeared into the seaweed.

A few shells shaped like one of the tents Granddad had that Grandma didn't know about were scattered across the rock, just above the Lup-lup. Cooper gave one of the shells a Lup-lup, then scrabbled it with his paw to try to see inside it.

"No," said Mama.

Cooper cocked his head. He had a feeling there was a Fwen inside the tent-shaped shell. "It must be very shy," thought Cooper when the shell didn't move.

After taking absolutely the best route—through the wet pool—to get back to Mum and Whisper, Cooper scooted to a halt in front of them.

"I made at least *three* Fwens," said Cooper to Whisper as they walked along. "An orange beetle, a fish, and a tent-shell."

"Wow, Coops, that's impressive," said Whisper, dragging Mum across the sand so that she could Snuff Cooper's paws and bottom.

When they returned to where the car had been parked another Snuff wafted through the salt and sand and fish. Food. Cooper's mouth watered hungrily. Surely, it was time for their three Chiplets?

Mum left to go to a little hut with a man inside in a funny hat.

Mama took both pups over to a table and poured Lup-lup into their bowl from a bottle.

Cooper was busy having the Lup-lup when he heard Whisper's tail thwacking against the wood of the table. What was so Wag?

Once he'd lifted his head, he agreed wholeheartedly that the situation was indeed extremely Wag.

Mum had brought two big boxes to the table. Both had steam coming from them, along with a Snuff so delicious and so strong that Cooper felt as though he would do Wees without meaning to.

"Oh my goodness, Whisp," said Cooper, his tail wagging so enthusiastically it hit both sides of his bottom, "the Chiplets have arrived."

"Whisper hopes Coops has been a Very Good Boy," said Whisper, seriously, "otherwise there will be no Chiplets for Coops today."

"Oh ya. I definitely have." He even did a very good sit and then a very good Beg to prove how much of a Very Good Boy he was.

Mum and Mama ate their fish and Chiplets far too slowly. Cooper knew he and Whisper wouldn't get any Chiplets until Mum and Mama had finished theirs. It was Woogle Law and Mum and Mama were law-abiding citizens.

Cooper was so excited. His tail swept the grass around the table and his paws flopped in the air when he did occasional Begs. Mum just patted his head and spoke to him in gentle tones. Cooper hoped she was reassuring him that he would be having Chiplets soon.

Finally, *eventually*, three Chiplets remained on Mum's plate and three Chiplets remained on Mama's plate.

Cooper went stock still, his eyes round, his lips parted. Air rushed in and out of his lungs as he sat in anticipation. If he'd been sitting on a chair, he would have been on the edge of it.

Mum patted Cooper's head and for a heartbreaking moment, Cooper thought she was telling him she was sorry but the three Chiplets were allocated for someone else. But then she said, "Good boy," and held one out to him.

Relief and happiness swam through him and made him gulp it down so quickly he barely tasted it.

Mum waited a little while before offering him a second Chiplet. Cooper made sure to take this one more slowly, savouring the taste and relishing how Wag it was to be given such a luxurious morsel of food.

He'd almost forgotten about the third Chiplet. He tried to pay the same amount of attention to it as he had the second Chiplet but, really, the second Chiplet had been the best one. No other Chiplet could compare.

Still wagging, Cooper licked Chiplet grease off Mum's fingers, much to her cries of disgust (which turned into laughter, so he didn't feel bad) and settled down at Mum's feet.

Whisper strained on her lead until Mama passed the lead to Mum so Whisper could be on the same side of the table as Cooper. With a sigh that sounded as Wag as Cooper felt, Whisper lay down next to him. "Whisper loves Chiplets," said Whisper.

"Ya," said Cooper, "I think they're probably my favourite things in the whole world."

"Yeah," said Whisper, "apart from biscuits."

"And Bally-ballys," said Cooper.

"And snuggles," said Whisper.

"And Swimmy-swims," said Cooper, "and Holly Bobs."

CHAPTER 11

Homeless

Once Whisper was back to normal, Old-Lady-Legs-wise, she enjoyed several energetic Walkies with Cooper. She chased his Bally-bally with him and sometimes she caught it and carried it around with her for the rest of the Walkies, proudly wiggling her bottom and running away if Mum or Mama got close enough to snatch it back.

The days were getting shorter and, very soon, it was dark well before Evening Wees and Sleeps. Whisper liked this time of year because it meant burying underneath lots of Blankies with Mum and Mama, flickering candles, and warm radiators. Mum and Mama stayed in more than they went out at home (as much as they were allowed to in the Dam Pendic) and many happy hours were spent cuddling on the big sofa in front of the Velly Tision.

After some especially energetic and fun Walkies where Whisper had stolen Cooper's ball for at least seventeen entire minutes, Mum was unclipping Whisper's lead when she exclaimed, "Oh no!"

Cooper trotted over, his feathery tail sweeping from side to side. "What's the matter, Whisp?" asked Cooper.

"Whisper's not sure," said Whisper, peering up at Mum. She put her bottom down and lifted her ears in a curious way.

Mum went away and brought Mama in to see. They both touched Whisper's collar and frowned at each other. Then Mum went out of the back door with a torch.

"Where has Mum gone?" asked Cooper, pressing his nose to the window. When he pulled away, he'd left a dirty smudge. He licked the glass, but that just made it worse.

"Whisper's still not sure," said Whisper and came to sit next to Cooper.

Cooper hopped backwards in shock and nearly fell over his own big, fluffy feet. "Oh my goodness! Look at your collar!"

"Whatisit?" Whisper tried to look at her own collar but the process of doing so was terribly awkward. Her eyes were simply in the wrong place to be able to do that.

"Your tag! Oh my Goodness!" Cooper ran about the kitchen, did some circles as he was prone to do when he was in a panic, and then stared at her. "Your tag isn't there anymore."

"Oh, Whisper's goodness!" cried Whisper. "This is not good at all."

With a tinkle of the bell on her collar, Dana ran into the room, chasing something neither of them could see. She swore in Puzzer language, then stopped to take in the two pups who looked like they'd seen a ghost.

"Dana!" cried Cooper, his tail down and his eyes round, "Whisper's tag is gone!"

"You puppies and losing things," said Dana, rolling her eyes. "Stupid, silly puppies." She used other words in Puzzer language that were too rude to repeat in pleasant company. "You know what that means, don't you?"

"No," said Cooper.

"No," said Whisper, half in a panic, half trying to remember when she had gone from having a tag to not having a tag. Even when she used all three of her brain cells, nothing came to mind.

"It means," said Dana, slowly, "that you are now..." She paused, an evil grin creeping onto her whiskered face.

"Now?" asked Cooper.

"Now?" asked Whisper.

"...Homeless!" Dana cackled her evil, Puzzer cat cackle and stalked away. Then she apparently saw the invisible thing she'd been chasing before and started off after it once more.

"Well, isn't Whisper in a pickle," said Whisper, her heart dropping.

"A right pickle, Whisp," said Cooper in a forlorn sort of way. "I suppose we shall have to build you a new house. I wonder if there are any bricks that someone doesn't want that we could use."

"Or," said Whisper, going to the back door again and peering into the darkness of the garden, "perhaps Whisper could live with Auntie Carol next door."

"Oh, how lovely," said Cooper, sitting beside her. "Auntie Carol does Wag cuddles and has special Biz Kits at her house."

"Yes, if Whisper must be homeless, Whisper reckons Whisper would prefer to be homeless with Auntie Carol."

"We shall pack your bags," said Cooper. He trotted over to the toy box and took out Whisper's Bee Hive. "Here is your Bee Hive," he said. He had his mouth full of Bee Hive, so it actually sounded like, "er is or ee ive."

"Thank you, Coop," said Whisper. She went into the living room to collect a Blankie. "Whisper will just take one of these as a carrying receptacle for Whisper's belongings."

"Shame we don't have any moving boxes, like when we moved home before," said Cooper after dropping the Bee Hive onto the Blankie.

They tried to wrap the Bee Hive in the Blankie to make a little pouch for Whisper to put onto the end of a stick, but every time Whisper picked up the Blankie, the Bee Hive fell out.

"Whisper's no good at being homeless," said Whisper after several attempts.

Cooper tilted his head to the side in thought. "Maybe Auntie Carol has toys and Blankies at her home. Whisper could borrow those."

"Good thinking, Coop," said Whisper. She sat in front of the door to wait for her official eviction letter and for Mum or Mama to tell her to leave.

Cooper spent a great number of minutes doing sorrowful sighs and little whines.

Mum returned from her excursion in the dark looking happy. Whisper thought this very odd.

Whisper was homeless; surely it was a sad time. Whisper was about to be evicted from living with Cooper and Dana and Mum and Mama. It was surely more miserable than the time she thought she'd have to go into an Old Woogle's Home?

Mum had something small and shiny in her hand. She went to put it under the tap. Then she undid Whisper's collar and pulled it from Whisper's neck.

Whisper went back to the door and sat, wondering whether Auntie Carol would allow her to be a homeless Woogle at her home.

But a moment later, Mum returned and reattached Whisper's collar around her neck. And Whisper's collar felt different. It felt heavier and made a jingling noise when she moved.

Cooper bounded over and snuffed under Whisper's chin. "Oh my goodness!" exclaimed Cooper. "Your tag has reappeared on your collar!"

"As if by magic," said Whisper in rather a lot of wonder.

"Ya." Cooper's tail bounced so excitedly from side to side he made a little wind. Either that, or he'd done a smell-less fluff. "I reckon I might have caused the tag to return with my Magical Wags."

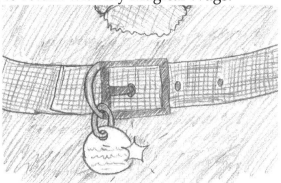

"Yeah," said Whisper, unsure what had made the tag return. She sighed. "Well, Whisper had better get ready to be homeless."

"No, Whisp," said Cooper, licking her ear, "you don't have to be homeless now you have your tag again."

"Oh, Whisper's goodness!" said Whisper, relief flooding through her. "Whisper didn't realise." She felt a hundred-and-seventeen times better than she had before and did a little spin to chase her tail in celebration.

Cooper nipped her back feet in an affectionate and brotherly way. "I'm so pleased," said Cooper.

Mum gave Whisper a big ear fuss before leaving the pups to have some Plays. And what Plays they had! Whisper felt like a new woman. She felt as if her freshly washed tag gave her extra Beans and she used those Beans to pick up Long Stick and waggle it in front of Cooper. He grabbed the other end and they had some Plays with that for a while.

Then they settled down on the floor to catch their breath.

Cooper put his chin on his paws. "Living with Auntie Carol would be very Wag," said Cooper. "She is very kind and fun. But I'd much rather you stayed here with me."

"Yeah," said Whisper, putting her own chin on her own paws. "Visiting Auntie Carol from time to time is just fine for Whisper."

"She does have good Biz Kits," said Cooper.

"Yeah," said Whisper, "but Auntie Carol doesn't have Coop, and she doesn't have Mum or Mama."

"Or Dana," said Cooper.

"Whisper wouldn't go that far," said Whisper.

Cooper just wagged his tail.

CHAPTER 12

Crispy Mouse

As the weather got colder, Mum and Mama seemed to be doing a lot of shopping. Every weekend they arrived home with bags upon bags of all shapes and sizes. None of the bags contained Bally-ballys, or Biz Kits, or anything else for either of the pups.

"Why are Mum and Mama buying so many things?" asked Cooper after a couple of weeks of stepping around bags he was not allowed to peek into.

"You see," said Whisper in a knowledgeable way, "an exciting event is about to happen. The event is called Crispy Mouse. It involves gifts, special music on the Velly Tision, and Mum and Mama wear very strange hats with white Bally-ballys on the end."

Cooper looked around the living room which was full of sparkly decorations. A large tree stood by the window adorned with pretty lights, shiny Bally-

ballys, and pretend birds. Mum and Mama had the Velly Tision on a noisy channel that showed people dancing in the snow and singing.

Mama was on the sofa. She had something fluffy in her hands that grew bigger the longer she held it. Attached to the something fluffy was some string which ended in a clump of fluffy stuff that unwound sometimes. Cooper tried to catch the clump of fluffy stuff when it jumped into the air, but Mama said, "No," firmly.

Cooper put his head on its side and considered the situation. Gifts were always a good thing, even if he wasn't the one receiving them. The shiny and sparkly decorations were a pleasant addition to the house and the tree smelled like forests and fun and frolics. Crispy Mouse must be a wonderful, exciting event indeed.

As the days went by, gifts appeared wrapped in patterned paper underneath the tree. Cooper Snuffed a couple of them but was told, "No," every time, so he just looked at them from the sofa. So far, he hadn't detected any Bally-bally-shaped ones, or bone-shaped ones, or any shaped like Biz Kits. He concluded that Woogles and Sprockerdors probably did not receive gifts at Crispy Mouse.

Auntie Carol came round for drinks one evening. She spent lots of time fussing Cooper's ears, and he spent lots of time leaning against her leg and enjoying her company. Mum and Mama were wearing jumpers with some kind of four-legged brown animal on them and making Auntie Carol lots of glasses of sparkly Lup-lup.

Mama went to the bag in which she'd been keeping the fluffy things that grew, and pulled two fluffy things out of it. She called Cooper over and stretched one of the fluffy things out before pulling it over his head.

For a moment or two, Cooper couldn't hear anything and the whole room went dark. "Who's turned off the lights?" asked Cooper, putting his paw up to push away whatever it was on his head. But

Mama fiddled with the thing and suddenly he could see again.

He concluded he was wearing a hat. He knew what a hat was because Mama and Mum wore hats sometimes when they did Walkies and it was cold or windy to keep their heads warm.

Mama pulled Cooper's ears out of holes on either side of the hat which meant he was able to hear properly again.

"S'lovely, Coop," said Whisper.

Mama pulled a similar hat onto Whisper's head, which also covered her eyes and ears, until it was adjusted. Whisper's ears, being smaller than Cooper's, remained inside the hat, which didn't have holes. Her hat had a fluffy Bally-bally on the end.

"So is yours, Whisp," said Cooper. His hat also had a white Bally-bally on the end of it, just like the hats Whisper had said Mum and Mama wore at Crispy Mouse. This was obviously a special Crispy Mouse hat.

Mum and Mama gave him lots of fusses, and then they gave Whisper lots of fusses as well. Clearly, they were pleased with the hats. Auntie Carol clapped her hands and made squealy-cooing noises at them, which meant she was pleased as well.

"Aren't we a fashionable pair?" said Whisper, sitting tall, her tongue hanging out in a delighted sort of way.

"Ya," said Cooper, "almost as fashionable as I look in my Fleshy Prince boots."

"Whisper reckons Whisper could be a fashion model," said Whisper, strutting around the room and wagging her tail, much to Auntie Carol's cheers.

"You definitely could," said Cooper, happy that Whisper was having a lovely time at Crispy Mouse.

If he was honest, Cooper wasn't all that impressed with the hat. The Bally-bally on the end kept smacking against his neck, and the entire thing continually slipped down over his eyes. Also, his floppy ears felt very constricted sticking out of the holes in the hat.

"As lovely as it is, I think I might take my hat off now," said Cooper, lifting a paw to dislodge the hat.

"But it is a Crispy Mouse gift from Mama," said Whisper. "You'd better be polite and keep it on. Otherwise, she'll think you don't like it and be very sad."

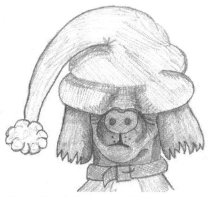

"Ooh," replied Cooper. He put his paw back on the floor and left the hat alone.

When it was Dindins time, which included a delicious combination of Meaty-chunks and Krunchy Kibble, presumably in celebration of Crispy Mouse, Mama took their hats off and put them on the kitchen table.

Cooper had a little dance once he was free. "Hurray! Now I can continue the evening in comfort."

"It'll just be during Dindins, Whisper expects," said Whisper with her mouth full. "Whisper's not sure what Coop is complaining about, though. Whisper *loves* Whisper's hat."

"Good for you," replied Cooper with a sigh.

After post-Dindins Ablutions, and as Whisper had predicted, Mama slipped the hat back onto Cooper's head.

Cooper considered shaking it onto the floor and point blank refusing to wear it ever again, but the joyful look on Mama's face and the way Mum cheered made him reconsider. After all, it *was* Crispy Mouse. And Cooper was a keen believer that happy parents were important and lovely things to have.

So there he sat, the uncomfortable hat slipping down every seventeen minutes so he couldn't see, the Bally-bally smacking his neck whenever he moved, trying to pretend he was, in fact, having a delightful evening.

Even when Dana stalked into the living room and cackled her Puzzer cat cackle at his hat—uttering a "Stupid puppy" as usual—Cooper remained bolt upright and loyally wearing his Crispy Mouse hat.

It became late, much later than Cooper would usually be allowed to stay up, and Mama and Mum and Auntie Carol developed red faces and sleepy-looking eyes. Dana had obviously had too much Nip as she was rolling about on the floor and exposing her white bloomers to the world, singing songs that contained words too rude to repeat in pleasant company.

Whisper had settled on the carpet with her chin on her paws, her own hat perched atop her head like a fluffy molehill. And still, Cooper remained sitting nicely and pretending his hat was the most comfortable thing he'd ever owned.

Eventually, it was time for Sleeps. Mum and Mama and Auntie Carol had started getting awfully silly—Cooper reckoned it had something to do with the fizzy Lup-lup they'd consumed in large quantities.

The pups were encouraged out for Evening Ablutions. Due to his slipped-down hat, Cooper stumbled into the garden, unable to see where the grass was. He had to rely on the tickly feeling under his paws and feet, and the grassy Snuff inside his nose. He did some Wees, then followed the Snuff of Whisper's wiggling bottom inside.

Getting into the kitchen was a completely different matter. All the floors Snuffed the same, and he couldn't tell where the doors were without the use of his eyes. When his journey was cut short by a collision with a wall that definitely had not been in front of him a moment ago, he let out a yelp. He shook his head vigorously, dislodging the hat so that it slipped completely over his head.

In total humiliation and misery, he sunk onto the floor, determined to stay exactly where he was in case he encountered any more unexpected walls. His forehead throbbed. "Ouch," whined Cooper, his voice muffled because of his entire head being covered in fluffy material, "I am in quite a predicament."

"It seems so," said Whisper sympathetically from somewhere close by.

Cooper could hear Dana laughing from the living room. He did another, pathetic, whine.

A soft hand rubbed Cooper's back. Mama's soft voice made its way through the fluff of the hat to Cooper's ears. Then the muffling, vision-impairing accessory was removed. Cooper blinked as the hallway came back into focus.

Mama was stroking his head and chuckling gently at him.

Cooper did a slow tail wag, unsure whether he'd been impolite or not. Was he in trouble? Perhaps it was okay that he didn't like the hat so much. Perhaps Mama wouldn't mind if he never, ever wore it again.

After giving his head a pat, Mama rolled the rim of the hat up and tucked the Bally-bally into the rolled up bit. Then she set the hat back onto Cooper's head but didn't pull his ears through the holes.

Cooper did another slow wag, which rapidly turned into a fast wag. That was *much* more comfortable. The Bally-bally didn't hit his neck when he moved because it was tucked away. The hat didn't slip down to cover his eyes because Mama had rolled the edge up. His ears no longer felt constricted because they weren't in the too-tight holes.

"Now, this is a hat I can get on board with," said Cooper, sitting upright and proud.

"Oh yeah, Coop," said Whisper, flopping down on the bed with a satisfied huff. Her own hat tumbled from her head a moment before being picked up by Mama, who placed it on the table. "S'lovely."

"It's lovely," said Cooper, his eyes drooping. It was, after all, much later than he would usually be allowed to stay up. It must be some kind of special Crispy Mouse tradition.

"Happy Crispy Mouse!" called Dana from the living room, although she inserted some words in Puzzer language into the sentence that were too rude to repeat in pleasant company.

"Happy Crispy Mouse, Dana," replied Whisper.

"Ya, happy Crispy Mouse!" Cooper stretched with his amended hat still on his head and settled next to Whisper on the bed.

"We had better get some Sleeps," said Whisper with an air of knowing, "otherwise Santy Paws won't come with our gifts on Crispy Mouse Day, which is tomorrow."

"We get gifts for Crispy Mouse that aren't hats?" asked Cooper, a sense of satisfaction settling over him.

"Oh yeah," replied Whisper, nuzzling Cooper's ear affectionately, "but those gifts come from Santy Paws, not Mum and Mama. Santy Paws arrives magically in the middle of the night with his Dears of Rain that pull a big vehicle much Poo-perior to Mum and Mama's car. Whisper almost always gets a new, shiny collar and some Biz Kits, which are Whisper's favourite thing. Whisper expects Cooper will get something that is his favourite thing too."

"How interesting," said Cooper sleepily.

"But Whisper and Cooper must have Sleeps, otherwise Santy Paws will not arrive."

Cooper pushed the hat from his head with his big paw and gave Mama a big-eyed look, just in case doing that wasn't polite. Even though the hat had been amended, he still didn't fancy wearing it whilst he had Sleeps. To his relief, Mama put it safely on the table with a soft chuckle. "Good boy," said Mama.

The hat wasn't so bad. Cooper would wear it all day tomorrow, on Crispy Mouse Day, so long as Mama made sure it was amended in the specific way that didn't make him walk into walls.

Cooper had Sleeps that were filled with dreams of walls that appeared out of nowhere, hats that appeared from Mum and Mama's car, and Dana receiving the biggest selection of white bloomers known to both Sprockerdor and Woogle-kind.

He was a very Wag boy.

Author Bio

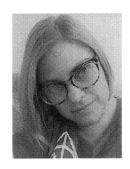 Squiz Gordon is the alter-ego of Jenn Matthews, a published author of contemporary romance between women. She lives in England's South-West with her wife, two dogs, and cat. When not working full-time as a healthcare assistant on a mental health rehab unit, she can be found avidly gardening, crocheting, writing, or visiting National Trust properties.

Inspired by life's lessons and experiences, Jenn is a passionate advocate of people on the fringe of society. She hopes to explore and represent other "invisible people" with her upcoming novels.

Catch up with Squiz at her website: www.jennmatthews.com

Woogle & Sprockerdor Lexicon

Ablutions General word for going to the toilet

Bally-bally/s Cooper's cylindrical toys

Beans Energy

(a) Beg A trick Cooper does where he sits on his back feet and flaps his paws in the air

Biz Kit Biscuit

Blankie Blanket

Bungled Burgled/robbed

Carer Coop A specialised job only Cooper can do

Cat-cophony A cat cacophony – loud commotion made by a cat

Choco-lit Chocolate, poisonous to dogs

Cooper Cuddle Specialised cuddle that only Cooper can do

Crispy Mouse Christmas

Daddy-dog	A dog's biological father
Dam Pendic	Pandemic; Covid-19 outbreak
Dears of Rain	Reindeer
Dindins	Dinner
Donut of Shame	An inflatable donut a dog wears around its neck to prevent him from licking a wound
Dreaded Washes	Woogle version of a bath/shower (Woogles are land mammals and don't like water)
Ducky	Cooper's soft toy duck
Flou-flou	Flower
Fluff-ectomy	A very complicated, medical procedure to remove the fluff from inside a toy
Fwen	Friend
Gubble Espresso	Coffee
Holly Bobs	Holiday
Hooman	Human

Hull of Soli	Solihull
iBone	Smartphone
Im-paw-tant	Important
(Krunchy) Kibble	Dry food
Lup-lup	Water; drink; lick
Magical Wags	A specialised wag only Cooper can do which has healing powers
Metty Cam	Metacam, a common painkiller for pets
Mummy Dog	a dog's biological mother
Nemesis	Vacuum cleaner
Nip	Dana's favourite treat.
Nip Night	Friday night, on which Puzzers consume nip
Nurse Whisp	A very specialised job only Whisper can do
Old Woogle's Home	Like an old people's home, but for Woogles
Paw-fect	Perfect

Pawly	Poorly/ill/injured
Pig Jun	Pigeon
Plays	Games
Poo-perior	Superior
Poopy-bags	Plastic bags taken on Walkies for collecting dog poop
Puppy-gate	Stair-gate
Puzzer cat	Dana's species
Retrieval Services	Playing fetch
Santy Paws	Santa Claus
Scrubby-scrubs	The act of rubbing in shampoo on a Woogle
Shakes	a full-body shake to get rid of water or an itch in the ear
Shampoop	shampoo
S'lovely	Woogle language for 'It's/that's lovely.'
Snuff/s	Sniff/s; smell/s
Special Puperation	Special operation

Sprockerdor	Cooper's breed; the language Cooper speaks (very similar to Woogle)
Spruce	Dog groom/haircut
Swimmy-swims	A swim
Tumbly	Rotund, chubby, overweight
Velly Tision	Television
Wag	Happy/good
Walkies	A dog walk
Wet Kibble	Wet food
Woogle	Whisper's breed; the language Whisper speaks (very similar to Sprockerdor)
Ya	Sprockerdor word for 'yes'
Yo-Goat	Yogurt
Zoomies	Where a dog (usually a puppy) has uncontrollable races, usually in circles

Printed in Great Britain
by Amazon